# 30 Days to SWIMSUIT LEAN

*From the national bestselling author of LEAN BODIES*

## CLIFF SHEATS

*and*

*Maggie Greenwood–Robinson*

TEAM LEAN PUBLISHING • FORT WORTH, TEXAS

TEAM LEAN PUBLISHING
1227 West Magnolia
Fort Worth, Texas 76104
(817) 921-9300

Other books by Cliff Sheats
*Cliff Sheats Lean Bodies*
*Cliff Sheats Lean Bodies Total Fitness*
*The Lean Bodies Cookbook*

Other books by Maggie Greenwood-Robinson
*Cliff Sheats Lean Bodies*
*Cliff Sheats Lean Bodies Total Fitness*
*BUILT! The New Bodybuilding for Everyone*
*High Performance Bodybuilding*
*John Parrillo's 50 Workout Secrets*
*High Performance Nutrition*
*Shape Training: The 8-Week Total Body Makeover*

Printed in the United States of America

ISBN 0-9653970-1-7

*Cover and book design by David Sims*
*Photography by John Dunn*

The suggestions for specific foods, nutritional supplements, and exercise in this book are not intended as a substitute for consultation with your physician. After you have met your desired body composition goals, it is recommended that you consult with a qualified health professional to establish food intake to maintain your energy needs. Long-term usage of nutritional supplementation is not recommended unless done so under the guidance of a physician, clinical nutritionist, or registered dietitian.

Individual needs vary, and no diet, nutrition program, or exercise plan will meet everyone's daily requirements. Before starting the Swimsuit Lean program, see your physician.

To Kathy, the wife of my youth.
It has been 20 great years of marriage!
Thank you.

# Thanks

This book would not be possible without the insights and talents of many people. My deepest thanks and appreciation go to:

Maggie Greenwood-Robinson, for exercising your limitless gifts of communication and motivation through your writing skills. As usual, you are a joy to work with, and excellence is your standard. My publisher, Team Lean Publishing, for their insight and direction in this project—especially Mark Hulme, John Dunn, Brenda Jones, and Bill Wellons. Also Margaret Allyson, for her careful eye and suggestions in the editing process. My great thanks to David Sims for going beyond the call of duty and for excellence in layout design.

Cindy Brinker, of Brinker Communications and Associates, for their professional assistance in getting this information into as many hands as possible. Wes Cade, for his valuable assistance in this project. His unrelenting eye for detail, knowledge in his field, and excellent people skills were most valuable to this project. John Parrillo, for his pioneering work in metabolic research. Crystal Littlefield and Marcey Berry, for lending their knowledge and talents to this project. Genesis Personal Training Center, for allowing us to photograph in their facility. I would like to thank BusyBody, America's Fitness Equipment Headquarters, for their support to this project. If you're looking for equipment, they are an excellent source. All the participants in the 30 Days to Swimsuit Lean program. They are heroes who inspire us.

My children, Allison and Jonathan, for being so flexible with Dad.

The Cokers, for their ever-encouraging friendship.

My Dad—special thanks to you for your continued encouragement and wisdom.

With all my heart, I would like to thank my Heavenly Father for His sovereign direction in my life and the privilege of working with such a great team of people.

*Cliff Sheats*
Dallas, Texas

# Contents

# III The Swimsuit Lean Workout

# IV Swimsuit Lean Maintenance

# Swimsuit
# Lean

# Chapter 1
## A Better Body—Fast

*D*o you dread putting on your bathing suit?

You're not alone. I know how you feel. I really do. In my Lean Bodies classes in Dallas, I've worked with plenty of people who would rather do anything but put on a bathing suit!

But once they learn how to get lean and firm the Lean Bodies way, they can't wait to strut around the pool or walk the beach in their bathing suits. They love their new shape, and feel good about themselves.

Wouldn't you want to have that kind of attitude—and more important, that kind of body?

You can. It's easy, and you can do it in just 30 days. That's all it takes.

If you're like most people, you've put off getting in shape. And now you wish you'd started dieting, exercising—or something—a lot sooner. After all, that vacation, high school reunion, cruise, or whatever you need to get in shape for, is just around the corner.

Good news: There's still plenty of time to make up for lost time. By following my 30-day Swimsuit Lean program, you'll transform your present shape into a lean, firm body. There's no guesswork involved either. I tell you exactly what to do each day for 30 days.

The best thing about Swimsuit Lean is that you don't have to deprive yourself of food. There's no crash dieting on 800 calories a day or less. You actually get to eat more food—not less—and trim down in the process. One secret lies in the kind of food you eat—food that is used to develop body-firming muscle, rather than to be stored as excess fat. Nor do you restrict caloric intake. Doing so only sabotages your fat-loss efforts, because your body starts producing fat instead of burning it. The more quality calories from food your body uses, the faster your metabolism—the body's internal food-to-fuel process. This all adds up to faster fat loss.

The other "secret" has to do with exercise. Unless you've been living on a desert island, you know that exercise has many trim-down/tone-up benefits. The problem is, most people don't know how to make exercise work for them. Has it ever seemed to you that it takes forever to see results from exercise? You won't feel that way on the Swimsuit Lean program. That's because you'll learn how to use exercise—both aerobics and strength training—to accelerate your fat loss. You'll also learn how to firm up troublesome body parts quickly. By targeting areas that need the most work, you can "restructure" your body—and do it rapidly.

To be successful on the Swimsuit Lean program, all you have to do is follow my exact instructions for meals and exercise each day of the 30-day program. Then watch the fat melt off—in just 30 days. That's an irresistible appeal if your previous attempts at getting in shape have failed.

But perhaps you're thinking: "Cliff, 30 days is a whole month. That's a long time!" Not really. Let's get some perspective here. If you're like me, you often wonder where the time goes. One day, it's summer; the next, it's winter. One day you're 30; the next day you're 40. Or so it seems. Time

## When you follow the Swimsuit Lean program, you should:

1. Find losing body fat to be much easier than ever before because this program will be more satisfying than any "diet" you've previously been on.
2. Have more energy all day long because you'll be fueling your body with high-grade food.
3. Firm up faster than ever before by using special combinations and timing of exercises.
4. Look great in your bathing suit —summer, winter, spring, or fall.

truly does fly. In the overall scope of things, 30 days is a mere speck of time to commit to a shape-up program.

Who says so?

About 30 people from all walks of life who agreed to participate in our initial Swimsuit Lean program and maintenance program. We recruited these people from the Dallas-Ft. Worth area to experience this breakthrough in fat loss. They overcame the odds and lost significant amounts of body fat in just 30 days. The proof is in their compelling stories and inspiring before-and-after photos that appear in this book. So powerful are these case studies and photos that any skeptic is sure to turn believer after reading them!

Here are several testimonials from our participants in their own words to provide you with inspiration—and proof that you can be swimsuit lean in 30 days too:

# Larry K.
## *A New Wardrobe Needed!*
At 217 pounds, I finally got sick and tired of feeling sick and tired, so I visited the Lean Bodies clinic to sign up for the Swimsuit Lean program. Prior to starting, I was very lethargic, easily winded, and could not bend over comfortably. I was eating lots of calories, but most of them were from fatty foods. I'd eat bacon and eggs for breakfast and chicken fried steak and mashed potatoes

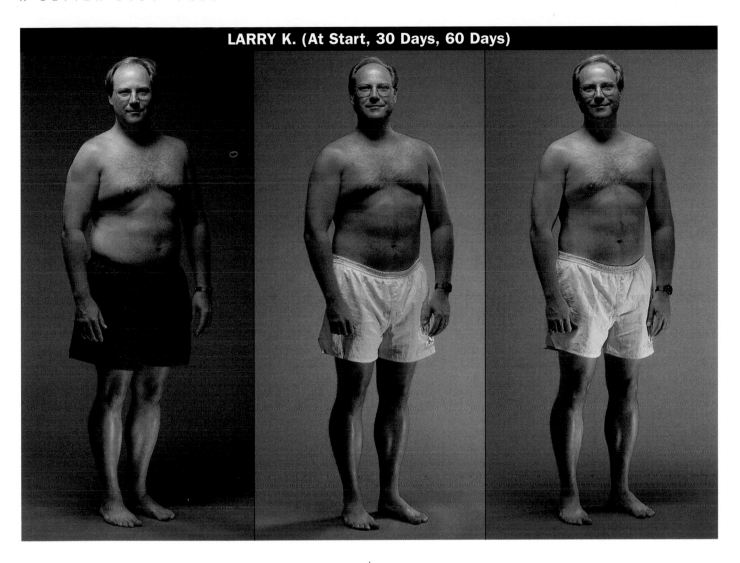

LARRY K. (At Start, 30 Days, 60 Days)

for lunch. Not until dinner time would I eat a healthy meal. I'd also snack on cookies, chips, and soft drinks throughout the day. I did virtually no exercise prior to the program, either. Walking the dog in the evening was the extent of my daily physical activity.

About two weeks before officially starting the program, I began to modify my eating. I started the 30-day program at 2300 calories and ended at about 2800. I no longer crave sweets and high-fat foods. My friends at the office were always commenting about how much and how often I was eating—and laughed at me when I'd complain about having to eat more calories.

At the beginning of the program, I resumed treadmill exercise (formerly engaged in, but later dropped) for 30 minutes a night for about four evenings a week. The second week, I added a 30-minute walk at 5 a.m. about three times a week. I soon built up to a 45-minute walk/jog five mornings a week and increased to an hour on the treadmill about four nights a week. I also added full-body strength training to my exercise program two to three times a week, usually right after work and before dinner. My endurance has increased dramatically, and I look forward to exercise. That's a big change for a veritable couch potato!

Including the two weeks prior to starting Swimsuit Lean, I've lost 17 pounds and three percent body fat in six weeks. I've trimmed at least two inches from my waist and chest. I need a new wardrobe! My collars don't choke me anymore. My face has a more chiseled look—not round and bloated—and is missing the extra two chins! My legs are well-defined, and I have bulging biceps. Lots of fat has melted from my upper body. I got out of the shower the other night, and my wife remarked, "Now there's the man I married!"

Mentally, I'm much more focused and get a lot more accomplished. My confidence has grown, and I'm happy with the way I look. I'm not making fat jokes about myself anymore. I feel fabulous!

# Nicole M.

## *A Tighter, More Toned Figure*

After having major back surgery, I lost all my muscle tone, and my flab was unbelievable. Plus, I had been a yo-yo dieter for years, always struggling to lose anywhere from 10 to 15 pounds. I started the Swimsuit Lean program to get in better shape.

While on the program, I increased my calories and ate five meals a day. At first, it was hard to do that. But now if I don't, my body tells me to eat five times daily anyway! As a result, my energy level has doubled.

Until Swimsuit Lean, my exercise history had been semi-consistent. I'd work out in spurts—six weeks very consistently, followed by six weeks of doing nothing at all. When I did exercise, I performed aerobic work only. Thanks to Swimsuit Lean, I work out five times a week with a combination of strength training and aerobics. Now I'm consistent, and I love working out. Best of all, I'm

getting great results. My legs are toning up, and the muscle definition in my arms has improved greatly. As for my back, my surgeon says I have recovered wonderfully and rapidly.

Over the 30-day period, I lost nearly four percent body fat—that's a lot—and gained five pounds of lean muscle. My clothes fit more loosely than ever. I feel great!

# Steven M.

## *He Finally Did It!*

Since graduating from college and getting married, I've gained a lot of body fat. I've tried every kind of "diet" there is, but each one only made me starve myself. Lost weight was quickly regained.

Before long, my suits became too tight, and my face looked fat. I saw myself go from a 34-35-inch waist up to a size 38. I told myself there was no way I could let myself get into the 40+ sizes. Still, for breakfast I would have two packages of doughnuts from the vending machine at work and drink colas all day long. For lunch, I'd eat fast foods or fried foods and dessert at a restaurant. By the end of the day, my wife and I were too tired to cook, so we'd order Chinese food or pizza or cook some kind of T.V. dinner. Being in sales, I felt there was no time in the day to eat healthy and exercise. Boy, was I wrong!

During the summer, my mother told me that Cliff Sheats was starting a "Swimsuit Lean in 30 Days" program. I knew this was the perfect opportunity to turn my life around and get healthy.

Wes Cade from the Lean Bodies staff took my weight and measured my body fat percentage. At 5'10" tall, I weighed 197.5 pounds, with 23 percent body fat. In my "before" picture, I looked like a short, stubby, fat, and out-of-shape person.

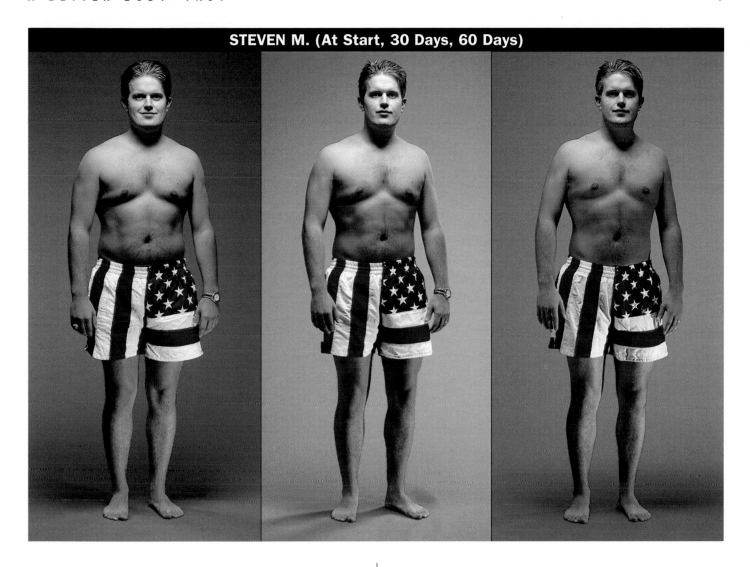

STEVEN M. (At Start, 30 Days, 60 Days)

Cliff helped me realize how much dietary fat I was consuming. Even though he didn't know me from Adam, he had faith in me—that I could succeed and look and feel great.

I couldn't believe that eating so much healthy food would help me lose weight. During the program, I had to work out and do some kind of aerobic activity. I knew if I could make it past the first two weeks, I could do the program for a month.

It wasn't until the third week that I noticed some big changes—and so did other people. My pants were getting looser, and my belt was pulling tighter. People in my office asked me what I was doing, that I looked skinnier in the face and that my clothes weren't as tight. Their comments and the changes I saw in myself motivated me to strive harder.

There was only one thing that bothered me. Every morning, I'd weigh myself. Over the weeks, I lost only a few pounds. I assumed something was amiss. But Cliff would say, "Don't worry about pounds or what your scales say. Be patient, and you'll see big results in the end."

And I did. By the end of 30 days, I weighed 192, and my body fat was 17.44 percent. I had also put on five pounds of lean muscle. Now I understand why Cliff said to not worry about pounds. When you lose five pounds of fat and gain five

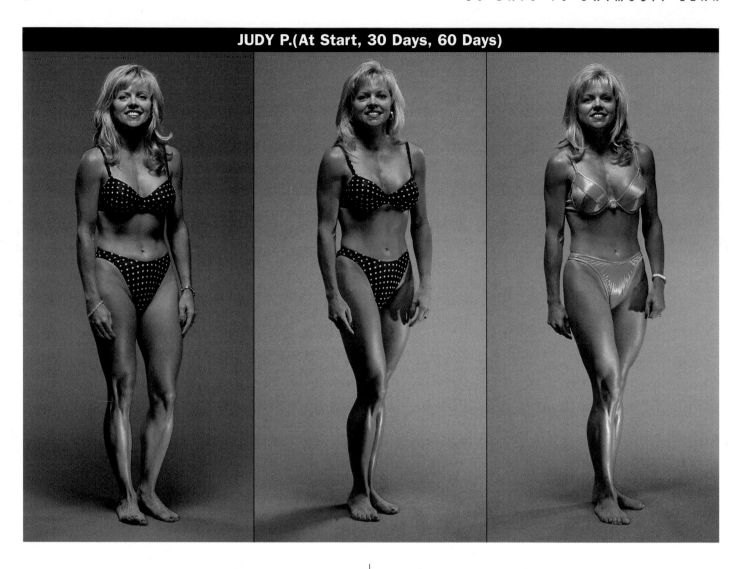

**JUDY P.(At Start, 30 Days, 60 Days)**

pounds of muscle, your weight won't change, but your appearance will—dramatically! Whoever thought a busy salesperson with no time could eat five meals a day, lift weights, do some aerobics, and actually lose body fat? I didn't believe it, but thanks to God, Cliff, Wes, my wife, and my parents, I finally did it. And I'm going to keep on doing it for the rest of my life.

# Judy P.

### *She Tweaked Her Physique*
Before I started the regular Lean Bodies program four years ago, I was eating around 1000 calories a day—and exercising! Lunch typically consisted of a diet cola, or nothing at all. Still, I wasn't making much progress. Participating in Lean Bodies taught me how to lose body fat and gain lean muscle by increasing calories. It worked.

With Swimsuit Lean, I wanted to tweak my physique—that is, get even leaner and gain a little more muscle. I began the program at 1600 calories a day for the first week, increased to 1700 the second, and finally leveled off at 1800, which is where I feel the strongest and most energetic. I run six to eight miles almost every day, but I had not been strength training. On Swimsuit Lean I added strength training to my exercise program four days a week. This change has made all the difference! I have much more muscle definition than ever before.

All in all, I lost 4 1/2 pounds of pure fat and gained 3 1/2 pounds of lean muscle. I continued to lose fat on the maintenance program, dropping another 2 1/2 pounds. I'm now at approximately 12.3 percent body fat, and I love my new muscle!

# Cary C.
## 16 1/2 Pounds Lighter

I'm a 44-year old real estate agent, business consultant, and father of two teenagers. My life revolves around business meetings, with a lot of time at a desk and in my car. I also try to participate in most of my family's activities, including ball games, choir rehearsals and performances, church activities, family outings, dates with my wife, and so forth.

My motivations for doing Swimsuit Lean were several. First, I needed to lose weight, probably around 25 to 30 pounds of fat. However, I did not want to lose any muscle weight. I also wanted to tone my body and lower my cholesterol level.

Many of my own sports activities have been curtailed, some eliminated, by a back injury several years ago. I'm no longer able to jog or play flag football, church league basketball, or softball. I've even had to cut back on other sports like golf and tennis.

Fortunately, though, both my doctor and my physical therapist have approved strength training as an exercise mode to complement my back therapy. I now work out regularly with a personal trainer. For aerobics, I use a recumbent bicycle at home four to five times a week.

The most significant changes I experienced during the 30-day period were a dramatic reduction in my waist size (from 42 inches to 38 inches),

a 16 1/2 pound fat loss (with no resulting loss in muscle) and more energy and stamina.

Many people have commented on my trimmed-down physique. My long-term goals are to continue to lose another 15 pounds, keep it off, and gain some additional lean muscle.

*Cary C. was one of the very first participants to follow Swimsuit Lean in its initial development stage. His body composition was taken by ultrasound.*

# Staci S.
## From a Snug Size 9 Pair of Jeans to a Comfortable Size 5

Prior to starting Swimsuit Lean, I felt fat, gross, and uncomfortable with myself. I've always had some kind of weight problem, bingeing and purging to control my weight. My weight continually fluctuated.

After going through a divorce, I stopped exercising and started going out to bars and drinking alcohol. I ate junk food all the time too. No wonder the pounds piled on so quickly. I gained more than 30 pounds in one year!

Now I'm eating healthier food as Cliff recommends and have lost inches. I can wear clothes that I once could not pull over my hips. Best of all, I have reduced from a snug size 9 pair of jeans to a comfortable size 5.

# Jerry M.
## I Can Wear My Wedding Band Again

I had been on the regular Lean Bodies program, which I started at 30 percent body fat. After about six months, I reduced that measurement to 21.64 percent. The Swimsuit Lean program gave me the opportunity to accelerate my fat loss, and I was successful in doing so.

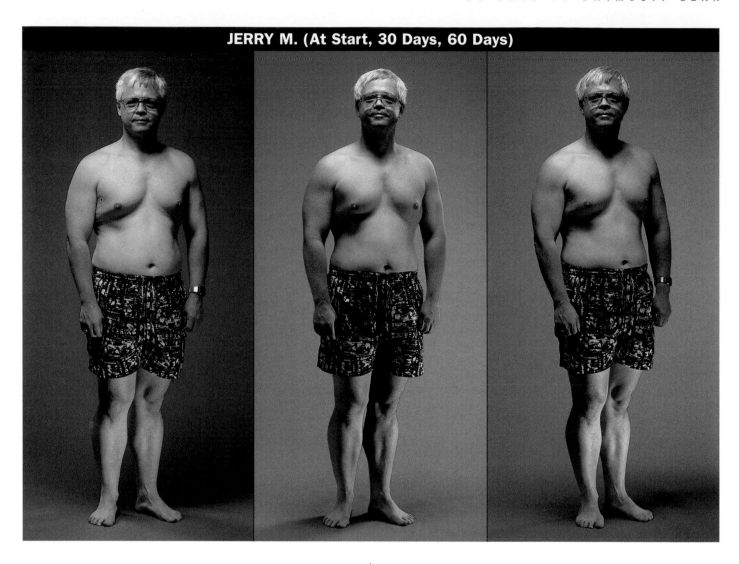

**JERRY M. (At Start, 30 Days, 60 Days)**

By the end of the 30-day period, I further scaled down my body fat—to 19.19 percent. I also dropped about five pounds of fat and gained more than two pounds of muscle—all while eating approximately 2500 calories a day. My total weight loss on Lean Bodies has been 25 pounds, and that includes six inches off my waist. It has been great to fit into clothes I haven't worn for a long time. Prior to Lean Bodies, I wasn't able to wear my wedding band because my ring finger got too fat. By the end of the 30-day Swimsuit Lean program, I was able to wear it again.

What helped me accelerate my fat loss was following Cliff's special recommendations for exercise timing, duration, and frequency. The hard work has paid off.

Exercise has been a major contributor to my increased levels of energy and better self-image. Because I look and feel better physically, I have a more positive outlook on just about everything.

# Syd M.

## *Following Doctor's Orders*

In 1994, I was diagnosed with Type II diabetes.* Then my weight ballooned to 299 pounds. My

*Individuals with Type II diabetes produce enough insulin but cannot process blood sugar properly.

doctor gave me an ultimatum: Take off your weight and bring your blood sugar down. So I started the Swimsuit Lean program.

I gradually increased my calories to between 2500 and 2800 a day. As a result, I was able to lose eight pounds of body fat and gain four pounds of muscle in only 30 days. Exercising helped reduce my blood sugar levels. I continued on Cliff's maintenance program and lost additional inches.

# Let's Get Started!

You don't have to take these people's word that this program works, although it's hard not to once you've see their pictures and read their stories.

The nutrition and exercise principles that form the core of Swimsuit Lean are all backed up by scientific research.

The Swimsuit Lean guidelines are spelled out in Chapter 10. In the chapters that precede it, you'll learn all about why this extraordinary program works and thus become convinced that Swimsuit Lean is the safe, rapid fat-loss program you've been seeking for so long.

Now, let's start getting swimsuit lean…

*To give the most accurate depiction possible of results, the photographs in this book were taken under consistent, controlled lighting situations. Due to logistical circumstances, however, not all participants were measured and photographed at the same time of the day.*

# Chapter 2
## *What to Expect in 30 Days*

*I*n the Swimsuit Lean program, we measure success in two major ways: first (and most important), by how many percentage points of body fat you drop; second, by the number of fat pounds you reduce.

While it might not sound like much, a reduction of a few points in body fat percentage can make a huge difference in how lean and firm you look. Just notice the before-and-after differences in Blythe F.'s physique on the next page. Her photos show what a five percent drop in body fat content can do for a woman's figure. So do the many other before-and-after photos that appear in this book.

Before beginning the Swimsuit Lean program, you should check your weight on the scales and have your body fat assessed. Scales will tell you the combined weight of your muscles, bones, body water, and fat. This is useful information, since lost fat will show up on the scales— but so will lost water weight and any muscle that you gain. A better measurement of how well you're losing fat is a body fat assessment. There are several ways to assess your body fat.

### SKINFOLD THICKNESS MEASUREMENTS

This method uses an instrument called a skinfold caliper to measure the thickness of a layer of fat just below the skin. For accuracy, between five to nine sites on the body are measured. The readings obtained from these measurements are plugged into a formula to calculate percentages of body fat and lean muscle. You should have your skinfolds measured by someone who is experienced in this technique. Ideally, the same per-

**BLYTHE F. (At Start, 30 Days)**

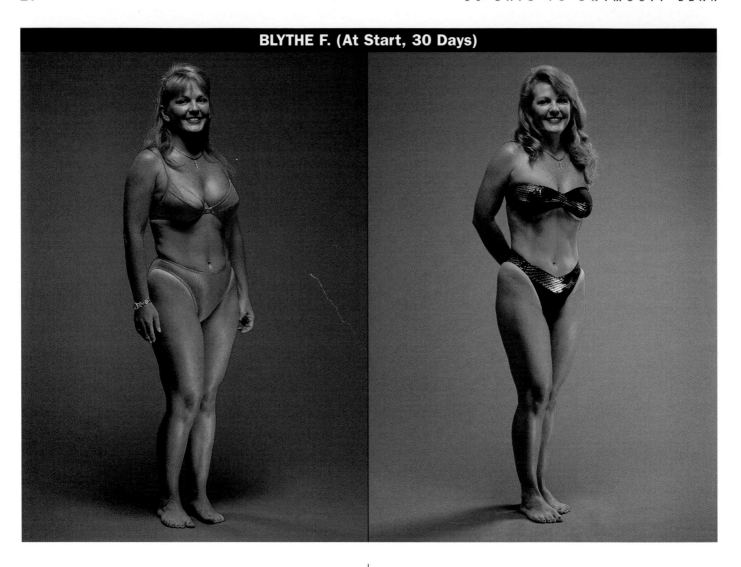

son should do the measurements each time. Many gyms and health clubs offer this service, either free or for a small fee.

## ULTRASOUND

Performed at your doctor's office or health club, ultrasound is considered to be a very reliable method of determining body fat percentage. Ultrasound waves pass through the skin and measure underlying fat and muscle. Scans are taken in several areas of the body, then estimated mathematically in a manner similar to skinfold thicknesses. This analysis reveals your body fat per-

centage in pounds, your lean mass percentage in pounds, total body water, and other important fitness measurements. Ultrasound is a simple, painless procedure that takes just five to ten minutes. The results are available immediately after the test.

## ELECTRICAL IMPEDANCE

This relatively new method of assessing body fat involves passing a painless electrical current through the body. It is based on the fact that body fat is a poor conductor of electricity, whereas muscle and body water are good conductors.

Therefore, body fat is easily determined by how fast the electric current flows through the body. The faster the current passes through the body, the less body fat there is. The current is introduced at electrodes placed on the hands and feet. Readings obtained from the test are put into special formulas adjusted for height, sex, and age to calculate body fat and muscle mass percentages. Many gyms and health clubs offer this kind of testing.

If you don't have access to these methods, there are other, less sophisticated ways to assess body fat. One is the mirror test. Simply look at yourself (without clothes) in the mirror and visually check the amount of fat on your arms, legs, buttocks, and abdominals. Though less sophisticated than the above methods, the mirror test can give you a quick "guesstimate" of how much of your weight is fat.

# About Your Fat Loss

Your body is constructed of different components. The largest components are water, body fat, and lean tissue (muscle). On dietary programs, weight loss reflects reductions in body fat, water, glycogen (the stored carbohydrate that fuels muscle cells), and muscle tissue. These may be lost at different rates and in different amounts.

The ideal situation is to lose mostly fat, while gaining or maintaining muscle. The Swimsuit Lean program, with its combination of caloric-adequate nutrition, aerobic exercise, and strength training, is designed to help you safely shed the maximum amount of body fat in the shortest amount of time.

It's not possible to predict weight loss precisely, even for people following the exact same eating plan or performing the same exercise routine. Fat loss varies from person to person, depending on activity level, motivation, present physical condition, and percentage of body fat and lean muscle upon starting the program. Nevertheless, everyone who follows this program to the letter will see results. The success stories of our participants are proof of that.

At first, you could lose weight rather quickly—perhaps three or four pounds. But this loss will be due to decreases in muscle carbohydrate and water reserves. As you progress on the program, carbohydrate and water losses level off. You'll still be losing weight, but on Swimsuit Lean, that weight is mostly body fat. And that's as it should be. A loss of 10 pounds of body weight may sound great, but if five pounds of that loss is muscle, you can still look less than firm. Plus, your energy and exercise performance could suffer.

On average, people on the Swimsuit Lean program can lose between one and two pounds of body fat a week. That's the safest rate of weight loss as recommended by medical professionals.

Some of you might wonder why you can't lose weight faster than that, get discouraged, and throw in the towel. Don't fall into this trap! Unless you understand what is happening to your body, the numbers you see on your scales might prompt you to quit. There are several reasons why you can't measure your progress solely by what your scales register. Most have to do with exercise, a vital regulator of fat loss on this program. For example:[1]

1 Exercise, particularly strength training, increases the size of muscles due to the growth of individual muscle cells. Pound for

pound, muscle weighs twice as much as fat. That's why you may even gain weight on this program. But it will be lean, body-firming muscle.

Keep in mind, too, that the muscle you develop is calorie-burning, metabolically active tissue. Having more of it revs up your metabolism and thus increases your fat-burning power.

❷ Exercise strengthens and thickens not only muscle but also connective tissue—tendons, ligaments, and joints. This slight but additional density can result in a small increase in body weight.

❸ With exercise, there is a build-up of energy substances in cells, particularly glycogen (stored carbohydrate). Glycogen binds with water, so at some point you may experience exercise-related water retention. On the other hand, hard-training exercisers may lose water rapidly during a workout—several pounds in fact. This loss is only temporary, however, and will return to normal after you drink some fluids.

❹ Aerobic exercise, in particular, stimulates an increase in blood volume (the amount of blood circulating in your body). In newcomers to aerobic exercise, this can equal up to a pound of body weight a week!

Remember that while all these body-weight components are being affected, your body is shedding the most important component of all: unsightly body fat. At the end of the 30-day period, when you have your body composition tested, you'll be pleasantly surprised by the amount of body fat you've left behind.

To help you see what to reasonably expect, I've broken down potential improvements into three categories. This information is based on our initial Swimsuit Lean program and the results we observed.

# 5 Pounds of Fat to Lose

You've probably read lots of articles on "losing those last five pounds." If that's your goal, Swimsuit Lean will do the trick. Judy P. lost her 4.5 pounds by following my 30-day program; that's a reduction of just over a pound a week—an average, safe rate of loss. But the best news of all is that most of those subtracted pounds were pure pudge! If you don't think that's a lot of fat, ask your butcher to weigh out five pounds of animal fat for you—or check out the picture in this book where I am holding a chunk of fat. Then imagine how much leaner you'd look in your swimsuit without that excess fat baggage!

# 10 Pounds of Fat to Lose

Many people emerge from their winter cocoons with roughly seven to ten pounds of extra fat. On average, that's how much you can gain between Thanksgiving and New Year's unless you're careful. Still, with Swimsuit Lean, it's possible to get rid of those unwanted pounds and be in near-perfect shape for summer. Other people start putting weight on by the end of the summer and need to get

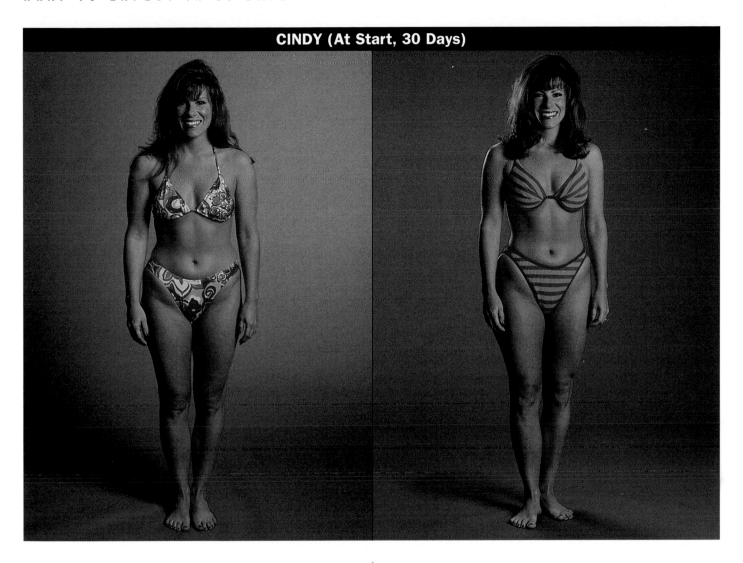

**CINDY (At Start, 30 Days)**

in shape for the holidays or a winter cruise. Swimsuit Lean can help you at any time during the year as long as you give yourself the allotted 30 days.

If you have around ten pounds to lose, you will see and feel results within the first week as your body starts shifting into a fat-burning mode. These positive changes will continue week after week as long as you stay true to the program. Expect to lose between one and two pounds of pure fat a week. As this fat is being removed, firm, defined muscles will begin to appear. You'll have more definition and shape than you ever thought possible. Plus, you'll feel incredibly energetic. A good motivator is to try your swimsuit on a few

mornings each week so you can check the visible results of your efforts.

## 15 or More Pounds of Fat to Lose

With Swimsuit Lean, changes begin right away. You will start feeling more energetic and stronger the first week, and by midway through the program, you should see a gradual diminishing of body fat. Early on, your weight loss should be fairly rapid, due partially to water and glycogen losses.

If you stick to the program perfectly—including the exercise recommendations—you may experience a fat loss of up to two pounds a week and a significant reduction in your body-fat percentage. By the end of the 30 days, you may lose 15 or more pounds of weight. A large proportion should be fat, along with some water and glycogen. Remember, rate of loss depends on individual factors.

Also, you should look much more defined—the result of diligent aerobics, strength training, and proper nutrition—as your much-improved physique begins to show through. If you have more fat to shed, you'll want to continue the program on a modified basis (see Chapter 20 for details) to reach your goals. This program works for everyone, no matter how much fat you have to lose!

# Chapter 3
## Anti-Fat, Pro-Health Nutrients

*I* call certain foods "anti-fat nutrients" because when eaten in the proper amounts and combinations, they help activate the metabolism so that the body burns fat more effectively. By including these foods in your diet, you actually help your body get rid of unwanted fat. The beauty of the Swimsuit Lean program is that you get to eat plenty of these anti-fat foods. Let's take a closer look at them and their many benefits.

## Lean Proteins

Found in every cell in your body, protein is a growth and maintenance nutrient. It is made up of sub-units called amino acids, which are reshuffled back into protein to make and repair body tissues. You get protein primarily from animal foods, although it is also found in certain vegetables such as legumes. Plant sources, however, don't contain all the amino acids needed for tissue-building. If you're a vegetarian, you must combine plant-based foods carefully so that those lacking in one amino acid are balanced by those sufficient in the same amino acid.

Protein activates the metabolism in two ways. First, high-protein meals can elevate the metabolism by as much as 30 percent above normal for up to 12 hours, compared to about 4 percent for a carbohydrate meal. With ample protein in your diet, your metabolism runs in high gear.

Second, protein is involved in building the most metabolically active tissue in your body—muscle. The more muscle you have, the more efficient your body is at burning fat. Adding just one pound of muscle to

| TABLE 3-1 | | |
|-----------|---|---|
| *Lean Proteins* | | |
| Amberjack | Lake trout | Sea bass |
| Bass | Longhorn beef | Shad |
| Bluefish | Mackerel | Shrimp |
| Chicken, white meat | Non-fat cottage cheese | Skim milk |
| Clams | Non-fat tofu | Snapper |
| Cod | Non-fat, no-sugar yogurt | Soybeans |
| Egg whites, cooked | Ocean catfish | Sugar-free soy milk |
| Flounder | Ocean perch | Swordfish |
| Game meats | Pike | Tuna |
| Grouper | Pollock | Turkey, white meat |
| Haddock | Rainbow trout | |
| Halibut | Salmon | |

your body helps you burn an additional 18,000 to 25,000 calories a year.

If you don't get enough protein and you're active, your body can start breaking down muscle tissue to get amino acids for energy. Consequently, you'll lose lean muscle and derail your fat-loss efforts. I think you can see why protein is an anti-fat nutrient.

On Swimsuit Lean, you're encouraged to exercise. That means you'll need more protein in your diet—for two important reasons:

❶ Exercise increases protein losses from the body in both urine and sweat. This protein must be replaced by the diet.

❷ Certain amino acids, namely leucine, valine, and isoleucine (the so-called branched-chain amino acids), help prevent the breakdown of muscle tissue during exercise. These amino acids are also selectively taken up by muscle cells and used directly in growth and repair. Your body can't make these amino acids; they must be supplied by the protein you eat.

The Swimsuit Lean program is moderately high in protein—to activate your metabolism and provide enough nutrients for growth and repair following exercise. All the protein choices on the Swimsuit Lean program are low in fat. That's important, because too much fat in the diet is both fattening and unhealthy. Table 3-1 lists your protein choices on the Swimsuit Lean program.

# Carbohydrates

Carbohydrates are foods derived from plants, and their primary function is to provide energy for the body. The body converts carbohydrates into either blood glucose, which circulates in the bloodstream, or glycogen, which is stored in the liver or muscles. Most of the carbohydrate stored by the body is in the form of muscle glycogen.

There are several reasons why carbohydrates have earned the right to be called "anti-fat nutrients":

❶ Their presence is required for the cellular processes involved in burning fat.

❷ Carbohydrate spares protein from being used

as fuel. The body burns carbohydrates for energy in preference to proteins. That way, proteins are spared so that they can be used to carry out their primary function of repairing tissue and building lean muscle.

❸ Carbohydrates from natural sources (whole grains, vegetables, and beans), rather than those from refined processed carbohydrates (cakes, cookies, sweets, etc.), restock the body with glycogen without triggering the release of too much insulin. (Insulin is a hormone that stimulates fat production, among other functions.)

❹ When the body is digesting carbohydrates, the metabolic rate goes up higher than it does when metabolizing fat. Whatever turns up the metabolism trims down body fat. As noted earlier, your metabolic rate is elevated the most by dietary protein, so when you combine protein and carbohydrates at each meal, as the Swimsuit Lean program suggests, you're really cranking up your metabolism.

# Starchy vs. Simple Carbohydrates

The main carbohydrates found in foods are starches, simple sugars, and fiber. The advantage of starchy carbohydrates (whole grains, potatoes, yams, legumes, etc.) in the diet is that during digestion they require prolonged breakdown and thus release glucose more slowly. This action helps maintain even energy levels and deters carbohydrates from being metabolized into body fat.

On the other hand, simple sugars such as honey, syrup, table sugar, and brown sugar release glucose very quickly. This triggers a surge of the hormone insulin. Insulin activates certain enzymes that promote fat storage (if your metabolism is slow).

Refined, highly processed carbohydrates such as muffins, rolls, bagels, and pasta are also problematic if you're trying to burn fat. These foods

---

## TABLE 3-2
### Starchy Carbohydrates

| | | |
|---|---|---|
| Barley | Bran ✳ | Popcorn, oil-free, air-popped ✳ |
| Beans | Bread - 100% stone ground ✳ | Potatoes ✳ |
| - Black beans | Bulgur wheat | Pumpkin |
| - Broadbeans | Corn, white | Rice, brown, wild |
| - Garbanzo beans | Corn, yellow | Rice, puffed ✳ |
| - Great Northern beans | Corn, sweet ✳ | Shredded wheat |
| - Kidney beans | Corn grits | Rutabagas |
| - Lima beans | Corn tortillas | Wheat germ |
| - Pinto beans | Cream of wheat | Winter squash, all varieties |
| - Red beans | Kasha | *(also a fibrous carbohydrate)* |
| - Soybeans | Lentils | Sweet potatoes ✳ |
| - White beans | Oatmeal | Yams |
| Beets | Parsnips *(also a fibrous carbohydrate)* | |
| Blackeyed peas | Peas | |

## TABLE 3-3

### Fibrous Vegetables

| | | |
|---|---|---|
| Alfalfa sprouts | Broccoflower | Spinach |
| Asparagus | Celery | Onions |
| Bamboo shoots | Collard greens | Peppers, green, red, yellow |
| Beans, green | Cucumbers | Peppers, hot |
| Beans, yellow or wax | Eggplant | Pimientos |
| Beet greens | Endive | Radishes |
| Broccoli | Kale | Summer squash, all varieties |
| Brussels sprouts | Leeks | Tomatoes |
| Cabbage, white | Lettuce - Romaine, red leaf, butter | Tomato juice |
| Cabbage, red | crunch, looseleaf, or bunching var- | Turnip greens |
| Cabbage, Savoy | ieties | Vegetable juice |
| Cabbage, Chinese | Mushrooms | Watercress |
| Carrots | Mustard greens | Zucchini |
| Cauliflower | Turnips | |

are easily changed into sugar in the body and thus very convertible into body fat. But don't feel disheartened about initially eliminating these foods. Once you reach your goal and are following my Swimsuit Lean maintenance program, you can start eating refined carbohydrates again.

If you like bread, you're in luck! You're permitted to eat bread while following the Swimsuit Lean program as long as it's 100 percent stone-ground bread. Many bakeries, local and national, make an excellent stone-ground bread that's sold at Kroger and other grocery stores.

Table 3-2 lists all the starchy carbohydrates you may eat on the Swimsuit Lean program.

# Fibrous Vegetables

Other types of natural carbohydrates included on the Swimsuit Lean program are fibrous vegetables. Low in calories, these vegetables are nutrient-rich and help fill you up without being con-

verted to fat stores. Table 3-3 lists the many fibrous vegetables you may eat on the Swimsuit Lean program.

# Fiber and Fat Loss

The starchy and fibrous food selections on the Swimsuit Lean program provide a third type of carbohydrate—fiber, the non-digestible portion of plant foods.

Fiber delays glucose absorption in the stomach and small intestine. That means glucose is released slowly, keeping your energy levels steady. Once it gets to the colon, fiber binds with or dilutes cancer-causing substances and ushers them out of the body.

A diet high in fiber will help keep you lean too—for several reasons:[1]

❶ Fiber makes you feel full.

❷ More energy (calories) is spent digesting and absorbing high-fiber foods.

❸ Fiber lowers insulin levels (remember, insulin is a hormone that stimulates fat production.)

❹ Fiber controls the appetite by stimulating the release of appetite-suppressing hormones.

❺ Fiber increases the time it takes for food to move through your system, meaning fewer calories are left to be stored as fat.

To get the protective benefits from fiber, the National Research Council recommends eating 20 to 35 grams of fiber a day.[2] With this in mind, it's a good idea to become familiar with the fiber content in foods. That way, you can make better high-fiber choices. Table 3-4 provides a list of Swimsuit Lean foods and the fiber they contain.

| TABLE 3-4 | | |
|---|---|---|
| *Fiber Content in Swimsuit Lean Foods* | | |
| **GRAINS & CEREALS** | | |
| **FOOD** | **SERVING SIZE** | **FIBER (GRAMS)** |
| 100 % stone ground bread | 1 slice | less than 1 |
| Shredded wheat | 2 biscuits | 1 |
| Brown rice | 1 cup | 1.6 |
| Bulgur wheat | 1 cup | 3 |
| **VEGETABLES** | | |
| **FOOD** | **SERVING SIZE** | **FIBER (GRAMS)** |
| Beans, kidney | 1/2 cup | 1.4 |
| Beans, pinto | 1/2 cup | 4 |
| Beans, garbanzos | 1/2 cup | 5 |
| Beans, lima | 1 cup | 3 |
| Corn | 1/2 cup | 4.7 |
| Lentils | 1 cup | 2.4 |
| Peas | 1 cup | 3.2 |
| Potato, white | 1 large | 1.2 |
| Yams | 1 cup | 1.8 |
| Spinach | 1 cup | 1 |
| Brussels sprouts | 1 cup | 2.1 |
| Carrots, cooked | 1 cup | 1.5 |
| Beans, green, cooked | 1 cup | 1.2 |
| **FRUITS** | | |
| **FOOD** | **SERVING SIZE** | **FIBER (GRAMS)** |
| Apple, Granny Smith | 1 medium | 1.8 |
| Strawberries | 1 cup | 2 |
| Blackberries | 1 cup | 5.9 |
| Raspberries, black | 1 cup | 7.65 |

*Adapted from Composition of Foods, Agriculture Handbook No. 8. Agricultural Research Service. U.S. Department of Agriculture.*

**TABLE 3-5**

# *Vitamin and Mineral Functions and Sources*

| NUTRIENT | MAJOR FUNCTIONS | FOOD SOURCES |
|---|---|---|
| **Vitamin A** beta carotene | Bolsters immunity, protective against certain cancers | Carrots; sweet potatoes; yams; orange, yellow, and red vegetables; green leafy vegetables |
| **Vitamin B$_1$** | Involved in carbohydrate metabolism | Whole grains |
| **Vitamin B$_2$** | Involved in metabolism and cellular respiration, required for the maintenance of healthy eyes, skin, and hair | Eggs, green leafy vegetables |
| **Niacin** | Involved in metabolism and the health of the circulatory system | Lean proteins and wheat germ |
| **Pyridoxine (B$_6$)** | Involved in carbohydrate metabolism and production of antibodies | Lean proteins and whole grains |
| **Pantothenic Acid** | Involved in cellular metabolism and health of the adrenal glands, essential for the synthesis of cholesterol | Whole grains |
| **Vitamin B$_{12}$** | Involved in metabolism, helps the body use iron | Lean proteins and dairy products |
| **Folic Acid** | Required for the formation of genetic material, involved in growth processes | Green leafy vegetables |
| **Biotin** | Assists in fat and carbohydrate oxidation | Rice, eggs, and legumes |
| **Vitamin C** | Maintains healthy gums, teeth, and capillaries; promotes the formation and health of connective tissue, enhances iron absorption, works as an antioxidant | Green and sweet red peppers, strawberries, raw cabbage, kiwi fruit, and green leafy vegetables |
| **Vitamin D** | Assists in the absorption of calcium | Fortified dairy products |
| **Vitamin E** | Involved in cellular respiration, protects against heart disease | Wheat germ, whole grains, polyunsaturated vegetable oils |
| **Vitamin K** | Necessary for the formation of a chemical required in blood clotting, required for normal liver function | Green leafy vegetables, polyunsaturated vegetable oils |
| **Iron** | Carries oxygen to cells for energy, involved in the formation of red blood cells, helps the body produce certain antioxidant enzymes | Lean proteins, and green leafy vegetables |
| **Calcium** | Builds and repairs bone, involved in muscle contraction and nerve transmission | Dairy products and green leafy vegetables |
| **Phosphorus** | Involved in metabolism and energy production, works with calcium to maintain bones | Lean proteins, eggs, and whole grains |

| TABLE 3-5 continued | | |
| :---: | :---: | :---: |
| **Vitamin and Mineral Functions and Sources** | | |
| **NUTRIENT** | **MAJOR FUNCTIONS** | **FOOD SOURCES** |
| **Selenium** | Works together with vitamin E in growth and metabolism, helps the body produce a key antioxidant enzyme | Whole grains, skim milk, lean proteins, broccoli, and onions |
| **Copper** | Assists in the formation of red blood cells and hemoglobin, required for metabolism, helps the body produce a key antioxidant enzyme | Whole grains, eggs, beans, and green leafy vegetables |
| **Magnesium** | Involved in metabolism, assists in bone growth, may protect against heart disease | Green vegetables, legumes, whole grains, and fish |
| **Potassium** | Regulates normal fluid balance, maintenance of normal growth, assists in the conversion of glucose to glycogen | Potatoes and other vegetables |
| **Zinc** | Involved in the absorption of B-complex vitamins and in metabolism | Lean proteins, oysters, mushrooms, and whole grains |

# Other Important Health Factors in Natural Carbohydrates:

## ■ *Phytochemicals*

When you eat the natural carbohydrates recommended on the Swimsuit Lean program, you're digesting a treasure trove of nutrients that have many disease-fighting properties—like "phytochemicals." Phytochemicals are plant chemicals found in vegetables, fruits, and grains. More than 40 have been isolated, and they appear to protect against cancer, heart disease, and other life-threatening illnesses.

There are thousands of phytochemicals in foods (tomatoes contain 10,000), many yet remain to be discovered. They exert their health-protecting action by various biochemical mechanisms, and the results are nothing short of amazing. Some examples:

### ANTI-TUMOR COMPOUNDS

In many cancers, tumors grow because new blood vessels leading to them are formed. Medically, this is known as "neovascularization." These new blood vessels thus feed the tumor with nutrients, allowing it to grow. If the formation of new blood vessels could be stopped, a tumor could literally be starved to death. Some promising news: Certain phytochemicals in soybeans appear to halt the development and progression of diseases associated with neovascularization.[3]

### CARCINOGEN INTERCEPTORS

Allyl sulfides, a group of phytochemicals found in garlic, onions, leeks, and shallots, also inhibit tumor growth. They do this by intercepting and breaking down activated carcinogens (cancer-inducing substances) before they can attack the genetic material inside cells. People who eat a lot of garlic and onion have lower risks of stomach and colon cancer, and allyl sulfides may be the reason.[4]

### ENZYME MAKERS

Enzymes are proteins your body makes to bring about various chemical changes inside cells. Vegetables such as broccoli, cabbage, Brussels sprouts, and cauliflower contain a phytochemical called sulphoraphane that boosts the production of anti-cancer enzymes. It works like this: Within a few hours after being eaten, sulphoraphane enters the bloodstream and begins circulating. Upon reaching the cells, it signals them to start making special enzymes. These enzymes detoxify carcinogens by attaching them to molecules that work like a conveyor belt. The carcinogens are then rolled right out of the cell before they can do any damage.[5]

### ESTROGEN COPYCATS

Plant protein foods such as tofu, soy milk, and other soy foods are packed with certain natural chemicals called phytoestrogens. Phytoestrogens mimic the effect of estrogen in the body and provide an amazing array of health benefits, including protection against cancer, osteoporosis, and menopausal symptoms. Soy protein has also been associated with a reduced risk of heart disease.[6]

### ■ Antioxidants

Natural carbohydrates are also loaded with health-preserving antioxidants such as beta carotene, vitamin C, vitamin E, and selenium. At the cellular level, antioxidants prevent "free radi-cal damage." Free radicals are volatile toxic molecules that cause harmful reactions in the body. In some cases, free radicals puncture cell membranes, preventing the intake of nutrients and thus starving the cells. In others, they tinker with the body's genetic material. This produces mutations that cause cells to act abnormally and reproduce uncontrollably. Dreaded diseases like cancer are often the result. In addition to cancer, scientists have linked some 60 diseases to free radicals. Among them: heart disease, Alzheimer's disease, arthritis, and cosmetic problems such as skin wrinkles. The cumulative effects of free radicals are thought to be the cause of the gradual deterioration we know as aging. Antioxidants guard against free radical damage and are thus health-protective.[7]

### ■ Folic Acid

Several starchy and fibrous carbohydrates on the Swimsuit Lean program are also rich in another nutrient now making news—folic acid, a B-complex vitamin. Found in green leafy vegetables, legumes, and whole grains, folic acid is necessary for a range of functions in the body, including the synthesis of RNA and DNA, the genetic material responsible for cell division.

Most of the excitement today over folic acid is being generated by its protective role against heart disease and cancer. The vitamin reduces homocysteine, a protein-like substance, in the tissues and blood. High homocysteine levels have been linked to heart disease. Scientists predict that as many as 50,000 premature deaths a year from heart disease could be prevented by increasing consumption of folic acid.[8]

Recent scientific experiments have revealed that folic acid deficiencies cause DNA damage that resembles the DNA damage in cancer cells.

This finding has led scientists to suggest a link between cancer and a folic acid deficiency.[9] Other studies show that low levels of folic acid appear to be associated with premalignant cell growth in the cervix.[10]

All the natural vitamins and minerals you need daily are found in the foods recommended on Swimsuit Lean program. Their functions and food sources are summarized in Table 3-5.

# What about Fruit?

Some people are surprised that in the initial weeks of my eating program fruits are limited to low-sugar fruits—Granny Smith apples, strawberries, blueberries, to name just a few. There are several reasons for this limitation.

Virtually all the calories supplied by fruit come in the form of simple sugars. Most of these sugars are fructose (fruit sugar), although some fruits (oranges and grapes, for example) contain a lot of glucose.

In the body, fructose can be fat-forming if you have a slow metabolism. Fructose has a different molecular structure than glucose and, consequently, your body uses it differently. During digestion, fructose bypasses a certain control point that decides if a dietary sugar is going to be stored as glycogen or deposited as fat. Most other natural carbohydrates such as rice, whole grains, and potatoes are preferentially stored as glycogen. But if not used first as energy, fructose is directly converted to fat in the liver. It is then whisked off to the bloodstream to be stored in fat cells.[11]

Fructose is also the major constituent of "high fructose corn syrup," a refined version of fructose made from corn and found in many processed foods. High fructose corn syrup appears to raise blood levels of dangerous cholesterol and triglyc-

| TABLE 3-6 |
| --- |
| *Low Sugar Fruits* |
| Blackberries |
| Blueberries |
| Boysenberries |
| Cranberries |
| Granny Smith apples |
| Green apples |
| Green pears |
| Kiwi fruit |
| Raspberries, black |
| Strawberries |

erides (fats in the blood and body tissues).[12]

As a nation, we're overdosing on fructose and the foods that contain it. Our per capita consumption of fructose, including high fructose corn syrup, accounts for more than 10 percent of total caloric intake. It's no wonder nutrition-related illnesses like heart disease and diabetes are on the rise. That's too much sugar for the human body to handle![13]

Fruits are extremely healthy foods and should be a part of your diet. But if you feel that your metabolism is slow or you want to maximize fat-burning, limit your fruit intake to moderate servings each week of either green apples or berries during the 30-day period of Swimsuit Lean. These fruits contain less fructose than other fruits do.

Table 3-6 provides a complete list of the fruits you may eat while following the 30-day Swimsuit Lean program.

# Dietary Fat

Of all nutrients, too much dietary fat seems to give us the most concern. This is because diets overloaded with fat (particularly animal fat) are

| TABLE 3-7 |
| :---: |
| *Essential Fatty Acids* |
| Borage oil |
| *(taken in capsule form - see usage recommendations on bottle)* |
| Canola oil |
| Evening primrose oil |
| Flaxseed oil |
| Hain All Blend |
| Safflower oil |
| Salmon oil |
| Soybean oil |
| Sunflower seed oil |

implicated in the development of obesity, heart disease, cancer, and other life-shortening diseases.

Nonetheless, fat is an essential nutrient and has many important functions in the body. You need some fat in your diet, but how much and what kind?

On the Swimsuit Lean program, your daily fat intake should not exceed 10 to 15 percent of your total calories. One of the main reasons for this low ratio is that too much dietary fat, like simple sugars, is easily converted to body fat. In fact, your body stores calories from fat much more easily than calories from carbohydrates. By a simple reduction in the amount of fat you eat, you can whittle away body fat, even while increasing calories from other foods.

The program, however, does not eliminate dietary fats altogether. Dietary fat, mainly from vegetable sources, is vital to health because it provides us with nutrients known as "essential fatty acids" or EFAs. These nutrients are linoleic acid, arachidonic acid, and linolenic acid. They keep your skin and hair healthy. They break down cholesterol in the body. They even help prevent other fats from being stored as fat—which is why even

these dietary fats can be labelled as "anti-fat" nutrients. EFAs can't be manufactured by the body. You must get them from the foods you eat.

To get the right amount of EFAs daily, all you have to do is eat two to three teaspoons of EFAs each day. Table 3-7 lists the EFAs you may eat on the program.

# Sugar Substitutes

Along with being low in fat, the Swimsuit Lean program is also low in sugar, designed this way to help you lose as much body fat as possible. But what if you have a sweet tooth? What's a body to do?

One option is to use sugar substitutes such as saccharin, aspartame, or acesulfame-K. Sugar substitutes, however, are controversial when it comes to weight control. In 1986, a study suggested that aspartame increased hunger by sending mixed signals to the brain, disrupting normal appetite.[14]

Since then, however, other better-controlled studies have been conducted, with quite different results. In a 12-week study at Harvard University, 59 obese men and women participated in a weight-loss program to study the effects of sugar substitutes. The study involved a moderately reduced calorie diet, exercise, and behavior modification. Half the people used aspartame-sweetened foods; the other half avoided aspartame. Both groups lost weight, but the participants consuming aspartame lost more weight (about one and a half pounds more) than those who used no aspartame.[15]

Most medical experts today agree that sugar substitutes help people follow their diets. One reason is that sugar substitutes give people more foods to choose from and thus make dieters feel less deprived.

My advice is to use sugar substitutes and the products they contain in moderation, since we don't know exactly what their long-term effects are. Even so, sweeteners and non-fat, non-sugar puddings and gelatins are perfectly permissible on the Swimsuit Lean program and are a good way to curb cravings for high-fat, sugary desserts. If you enjoy desserts, see the recipe at right that has been popular among other dessert lovers in our Lean Bodies program.

# Fat-Replacers

Food scientists have long been at work developing a suitable substitute for dietary fat—one that tastes good but doesn't produce any of the bad health effects of real fat. The most recent of these synthetic fats is olestra, now being used in snack chips. Olestra is derived from sugar and vegetable oil. Unlike other fat replacers, it tastes like real, honest-to-goodness fat. Structurally, its molecules are so large and tightly packed that the body can't break it down. Thus, olestra passes out of the body undigested, destined never to turn into artery-clogging and waist-clinging fat.

Critics of olestra say that it acts like a laxative, depleting the body of important nutrients such as beta carotene and vitamins A and K. The vitamins supposedly attach themselves to olestra and thus get flushed out of the body. The maker of olestra vigorously defends the product against its critics, but interestingly enough, plans to fortify the fat replacer with vitamins.[16]

It may be too early to tell who's right or wrong in the fat-replacer debate. My position on food has always been to select foods that are as close as possible to the way God made them. Man-made products—sugar substitutes and fat replacers included—are simply not used as efficiently by the

## Swimsuit Lean Dessert Crepes

*Crepes:*
In a mixing bowl, combine
**1 cup oatmeal flour**
  *(ground from oatmeal flakes in your blender)*
**1 1/2 cups skim milk**
**2 egg whites**
**Salt substitute to taste.**

Beat with a rotary beater until blended. Heat a non-stick 6-inch skillet and lightly spray with vegetable cooking spray. Remove from heat. Spoon about 3 tablespoons of batter into skillet. Lift and tilt skillet to spread batter. Return to heat. Brown only on one side. Invert pan over paper towel and remove crepe. Repeat to make about 10 crepes. (To freeze, stack crepes between layers of waxed paper. Freeze up to four months. Thaw before using.)

*Filling:*
**Instant non-fat sugar-free vanilla pudding**
**Fresh strawberries or blueberries**

Prepare instant non-fat sugar-free vanilla pudding according to package directions. Wash and drain fresh strawberries or blueberries. Reserve a small portion of pudding; add berries to remaining pudding and stir. Place about 1/4 cup of this mixture on each crepe and roll up. Drizzle reserved pudding on top and place one berry as a garnish on top of crepe. Enjoy!

body and may produce some unwelcome and untoward health reactions.

# Condiments

Because you won't be eating foods swimming in butter, buttery sauces, or fat-laced salad dressings, you may want to pep up your meals with condiments. Here's a list of condiments and flavorings you may use on the Swimsuit Lean program:

- All sugar-free and fat-free spices and herbs
- Orange or lemon zest
- Butter seasonings such as Molly McButter

- Flavorings and extracts
- Sugar substitutes (in moderate amounts)
- Mustard
- Sugar-free ketchup
- Lite barbecue sauce
- Vinegar
- Lemon juice
- Lime juice
- Soy sauce (preferably "lite")
- Worcestershire sauce
- Liquid smoke
- Fat-free salad dressings

# Chapter 4
## Anti-Fat Supplements

*N*ot long ago, a Gallup Survey revealed that 38 percent of all adults take vitamin and mineral supplements. Of this group, 84 percent take supplements every day.[1] There are many reasons why people supplement, but for the most part, they use supplements as a nutritional insurance policy to fill in the gaps against potential dietary omissions. That's a use I support. It's an excellent idea to take a vitamin/mineral supplement daily, preferably an antioxidant formula containing the nutrients beta carotene, vitamin C, vitamin E, and selenium.

As I mentioned in the previous chapter, antioxidants defend the body against harmful molecular wastes called free radicals. Free radicals are generated by metabolism, stress, sunlight, exposure to environmental pollutants, respiration—and even exercise.

During exercise, the production of these biochemical troublemakers is accelerated as your body processes more oxygen. In fact, when you exercise vigorously, your lungs use oxygen at 10 to 20 times your normal rate of breathing. The more oxygen you use, the more free radicals your body creates. Fortunately, eating lots of antioxidant-rich foods and supplementing with antioxidants helps protect your body against exercise related free radical damage.[2]

Keep in mind though: Nutritional supplements should never replace a proper diet. We would all benefit more from a healthier selection of foods than from taking more supplements. In fact, many of the nutritional problems that plague us today—including overweight and obesity—are not always vitamin and mineral deficiencies; they are problems related to eating foods that are over-processed, high in fat and cholesterol, and low in fiber.

I want to emphasize at the outset: You do not have to take nutritional supplements to be successful on the Swimsuit Lean program. Foods, not supplements, should be your major source of nutrients. You'll still lose body fat on this program, whether or not you use supplements.

Even so, there are some supplements that make the Swimsuit Lean program easier and more convenient to follow. These include sports nutrition bars, carbohydrate supplements, and protein powder, all used as part of your "mock meals"—the two extra meals you get to eat every day. (For information on mock meals, see Chapter 6.)

Two other supplements—lipotropics and creatine monohydrate—have special benefits that may make it easier for you to shed body fat and stay lean. Another supplement, MCT oil, is an excellent way to add calories to your diet and thus gain extra energy.

I call these supplements "anti-fat supplements" because they're designed to work with the Swimsuit Lean program to ensure that your body has everything it needs to burn fat at peak efficiency. None are miracle workers, however. If you're overweight and the only change you make in your lifestyle is to take these supplements, nothing will happen. You have to make major improvements in your diet and become more active by exercising regularly. These optional supplements are discussed next.

## ■ *Sports Nutrition Bars*

These are candy-bar-like products that contain low-fat protein and complex carbohydrates. Convenient to pack in a gym bag or purse, these bars are an excellent way to gradually increase your calories for a metabolic boost. On the Swimsuit Lean program, you can make the bar your "mock-meal" between breakfast and lunch, or between lunch and dinner.

Cary C., who lost 16 1/2 pounds on the Swimsuit Lean program, kept these bars in his car, briefcase, and at home. "The bars made it easy to get in my extra two meals a day, without much fuss or preparation. Plus, they helped keep my energy levels up at mid-morning and mid-afternoon," he said.

For a recommended sports nutrition bar to use on the Swimsuit Lean program, see Appendix A.

## ■ *Carbohydrate Supplements*

Carbohydrate supplements can also be used to concoct a mock meal. The best product to use is one containing maltodextrin as the sole or primary carbohydrate. Derived from corn, maltodextrin is a type of "glucose polymer." A glucose polymer is a chain of glucose molecules that is shorter than starch but longer than simple sugars. This molecular make-up gives maltodextrin "slow-release" characteristics. In other words, it breaks down more slowly than simple sugars, producing a more moderate insulin reaction and a more uniform energy level. Consequently, maltodextrin is not so likely to be converted to fat. For a list of the carbohydrate supplements recommended on the Swimsuit Lean program, see Appendix A.

## ■ *Protein Powder*

Protein powders can also be used as part of your mock meal, eaten with a carbohydrate or mixed in with a carbohydrate supplement (see Appendix A for recommended products).

The combination of protein and carbohydrates in supplement form can give you a real advantage while following the Swimsuit Lean program. As I explained in Chapter 3, a combined meal of protein and carbohydrates elevates your metabolism—and that means a greater fat-burning potential.

Here's a recipe that shows you how to combine carbohydrate and protein supplements in a single delicious shake:

## Cliff's Cooler

8 ice cubes
1/2 cup water
1 scoop of carbohydrate supplement
1 scoop of protein powder
1/2 scoop sugar-free chocolate powder
1/2 tsp. vanilla extract
Combine the above ingredients in a blender, and blend until thick and frothy.

## ■ *Lipotropic Supplements*

Lipotropic supplement formulas contain various nutrients involved in fat mobilization. Some of the key nutrients are L-carnitine, chromium picolinate, choline, and inositol.

One of the most extensively studied sports supplements, L-carnitine is a vitamin-like nutrient that shuttles fat inside cells to be burned. Several studies have shown that carnitine supplementation boosts oxygen consumption (which is a measure of energy production and metabolic rate), increases fat utilization during exercise, and enhances exercise performance.[3]

Another nutrient in many lipotropic formulations is chromium picolinate, a mineral involved in the metabolism of carbohydrates and fat for energy. Dietary shortfalls of chromium intake are very common. What's more, exercise can increase chromium losses from the body.[4]

Some evidence exists that chromium may be involved in stimulating lean body mass in people who strength train. A study of 31 college football players taking 200 mcg a day of chromium for six weeks, while strength training, lost an average of 2.7 percent body fat and gained 1.8 kg of lean muscle mass.[5]

The jury is still out as to whether chromium plays a possible role in muscle gains. Common sense would say that those who are deficient in chromium may experience some effect.

The liver requires choline to metabolize certain fats and to make "acetylcholine," a substance in the nerves that triggers muscle contractions. Limited amounts of choline are made by the body. Without enough choline, fat accumulates in the liver and cannot be transported to muscle cells to be burned. Like choline, inositol also helps the liver metabolize fat, and a deficiency can result in fat build-up in the liver.

Two other lipotropics typically found in these supplements include betaine, a substance from which choline is formed; and methionine, an amino acid that, like choline, helps mobilize fat.

**Important:** If you decide to supplement with a lipotropic formula, follow the manufacturer's suggestion for usage. See Appendix A for recommended products with which we've had good results at our clinic.

## ■ *Creatine Monohydrate*

Creatine is a constituent of muscles that assists in the transfer of energy in muscle cells and in the production of ATP, a molecular fuel that powers muscular contractions. Creatine is found naturally in red meat.

Creatine is available as a nutritional supplement known as creatine monohydrate. Loading your muscles with supplemental creatine accelerates energy production in muscle cells. This muscular energy boost helps you work out longer and harder when you strength train. The ultimate result is better muscular development and improved strength. As you gain extra muscle and thus increase your metabolism, you can ultimately burn more body fat. So indirectly, creatine assists in losing body fat and gaining lean muscle.

My co-author, Maggie Greenwood-Robinson, related the following story to me: Her husband Jeff was sitting with his arms folded during dinner at a restaurant one evening when some friends remarked, "Look at Jeff's biceps. They've gotten so big!" A true observation—Jeff had been supplementing with creatine for about six months and making huge jumps in his strength training poundages as a result. For the first time in years, he had experienced a substantial growth spurt.

Creatine monohydrate is nontoxic. The only known side effect is stomach upset if you take too much at once. Follow the manufacturer's recommendation for usage. See Appendix A for recommended products.

### ■ *MCT Oil*

Often called the "fatless fat," this cholesterol-free vegetable oil is a very concentrated source of calories that can be used for energy. MCT (medium chain triglycerides) oil is burned so quickly that its calories are turned into body heat—a reaction that boosts the metabolic rate. For this reason, MCTs rarely end up being stored as body fat.

Also, during a series of energy-producing reactions inside cells, a large portion of MCTs is converted into substances called "ketones," which are by-products of fat metabolism. If not excreted, ketones are used by muscles for fuel—a process that spares carbohydrates for more sustained energy.

Available in health food stores or sports nutrition centers, MCT oil tastes delicious when used as a salad dressing or drizzled on vegetables. You can even cook with it.

Gradually introduce MCT oil into your diet at the rate of a few teaspoons a day. This supplement is so rapidly absorbed that it tends to cause stomach cramping if too much is taken at one time or on an empty stomach.

As with any supplement, you should consult your physician before taking MCT oil. This is especially true for diabetics, individuals with a condition called ketosis, or women who are pregnant or lactating. Consult your physician. See Appendix A for recommended products.

# Questionable Anti-Fat Supplements

Many people have asked me about "thermogenic formulas" that reportedly boost the metabolism and help burn fat. These formulas contain the Chinese herb ephedra or an extract of kola nut. Ephedra is a stimulant from which the cold remedy drugs ephedrine and pseudoephedrine are synthesized. I advise against using any supplement containing ephedra since it can produce serious central nervous system side effects such as agitation, sleeplessness, and anxiety. People with heart disease and high blood pressure should definitely stay away from ephedra.[6]

Kola nut extract contains caffeine and thus should not be taken by anyone who has been medically advised to avoid caffeine and caffeine-containing products. Anyone with high blood pressure, heart disease, thyroid problems, or who is pregnant or lactating should avoid any supplement formulated with kola nut.[7]

# Chapter 5

## *Calories—How High Can You Go?*

In the same way a tablespoon measures volume, a "calorie" measures energy—specifically the amount of energy stored in carbohydrates, proteins, and fats. All foods supply calories, but some contain more than others. Fats have the most, about 9 calories per gram, and carbohydrates and proteins supply about 4 calories per gram. The caloric value of a large baked potato, for example, comes from the 32 grams of carbohydrate, the 4 grams of protein, and the 1.2 grams of fat it contains:

| | |
|---|---|
| 32 grams carbohydrate x 4 calories per gram = 128 | calories |
| 4 grams protein x 4 calories per gram = 16 | calories |
| 1.2 grams fat x 9 calories per gram = 10.8 | calories |
| **Total calories = 154.8 calories** | |

Most reducing diets are based on restricting the amount of calories consumed, typically to 1200 calories a day or under. That's a sub-par requirement, particularly for women. Here's why: An average woman's basal metabolic rate (BMR) is 1200 calories a day. BMR refers to the minimum number of calories required by the body over a 24-hour period just to breathe, to pump blood through the circulatory system, and to drive all the cellular processes that support life. The BMR doesn't include the energy needed to do other things like move around or exercise. So you see: Most diets are too low to provide enough energy to sustain vital functions, let alone other activities. Thus, the metabolism downshifts greatly.

With diets that are too restrictive in calories, the dieter at first experiences a rather quick drop in weight, but this loss is mostly water and stored carbohydrate, not body fat. Later some fat will be lost, but along with it, muscle tissue (including heart muscle).

It's estimated that restrictive diets cause a 3 to 6 percent loss of muscle tissue. If you go off such a diet and regain weight, that weight will be mostly fat, not muscle.[1]

The misperception exists that the fewer calories you eat, the faster you will lose weight, and the more weight you will lose. The results of an intriguing scientific experiment prove otherwise. Researchers at the University of Pennsylvania and Syracuse University put 76 obese women on one of three diets—a 420-, 660-, or 800-calorie-a-day diet. Basically, the dieters consumed a specially formulated liquid supplement. The experiment lasted six months, and all the women lost weight—an average of 45 pounds. There wasn't much difference in the amount or rate of loss among the three groups, either. But here's the clincher: These women lost weight at the rate of just under two pounds a week—what most weight loss experts call a safe rate of loss.[2] But they did it under near-starvation conditions! On Swimsuit Lean, you can get the same results on a low-fat, nutrient-rich diet—without slashing calories so severely, without depriving yourself, and without slowing down your metabolism!

Most dieters are rollercoaster dieters; that is, they go on and off diets. Even this diet pattern doesn't produce results! In one scientific study, researchers surveyed a group of women who were chronic on-again, off-again dieters. They learned that even though the women's weight fluctuated daily and weekly, they hadn't lost an ounce of weight over a six-month period.[3]

In the process of restrictive dieting, the metabolism decelerates considerably—for two reasons. First, the metabolic rate slows down to conserve energy and accommodate the lower calorie intake. Second, muscle is lost. Since muscle is the body's major metabolically active tissue, losing it compromises the ability of the body to effectively burn energy. It becomes increasingly difficult for the body to burn fat under these circumstances. In fact, the body starts thinking it's starving and begins hoarding fat, rather than burning it. The whole cut-calorie approach to fat loss is self-defeating.

Clearly, restrictive dieting fails to produce any meaningful fat loss. Not only that, there are some serious psychological repercussions to cutting back on your eating. In a famous World War II study, normal-weight men were asked to restrict their food intake for six months to lose 25 percent of their body weight so that researchers could study the effects of semi-starvation on the body. Their goal was to use the findings to learn how to treat the starving survivors of concentration camps in Europe.

In six months, the men lost an average of 50 pounds. The psychological reactions that emerged were startling. The men became increasingly obsessed with food. They collected recipes, pinned up pictures of food on their walls, even pursued food-related careers such as becoming a chef. Emotionally, the men turned irritable, upset, and combative. One subject was quoted as saying: "We lost our semblance of humanity and became similar to beasts."[4]

What's more, the subjects turned apathetic and lost interest in sex. And once the men were allowed to resume normal eating, they tended to binge on food. In other words, food restriction turned normal eaters into binge eaters.[5]

Other scientific studies of the psychological effects of food deprivation report strikingly similar findings. Food-deprived people—restrictive dieters included—tend to experience anxiety, low self-esteem, mood swings, depression, and irritability. Plus, they're more apt to indulge in binge behavior.[6] What a downer! Life can be stressful enough—why introduce another stressor (restrictive dieting) into the mix?

# Fat Burning with Increased Calories

Among the best ways to shift the body into a fat-burning mode is to add more calories. Gradually increasing calories recharges the metabolism so that the body can better burn fat for energy.

Of course, if you increase calories from the wrong kinds of foods, you'll store those calories as fat. One of the most significant factors influencing fat gain is the source of calories consumed. An excess of fat calories, for example, is likely to be stored as body fat.

In one study, researchers compared the fat intake of 205 women to their body-fat percentages as measured by skinfold calipers. The women filled out questionnaires about their diets, exercise habits, and lifestyles. An analysis of the questionnaires revealed that the most significant predictor of fatness was fat in the diet.[7]

As I described in Chapter 3, your body uses more energy to break down protein and carbohydrates than it uses to metabolize fat. Because dietary fat chemically resembles body fat, very little energy is required to process it. Instead, it heads straight to storage.

Too much sugar is just as bad. In a study at Indiana University in Bloomington, researchers analyzed the diets of four groups of people: lean men (average body fat 15 percent), lean women (average body fat 20 percent), obese men (average body fat 25 percent), and obese women (average body fat 35 percent). Those who were obese ate more of their calories from fat (as high as 36 percent of total calories) and simple sugars such as candy, doughnuts, and ice cream, which are also high in fat.[8]

Why the correlation? One reason is that too much refined sugar can cause the body to over-produce the hormone insulin, a reaction that sets fat production in motion.

The message here is that excess dietary fat and sugary foods can make you fat. Steer clear of them if you want to get lean. As I pointed out in Chapter 3, the Swimsuit Lean program is designed around anti-fat foods—foods that are not likely to be stored as surplus body fat. While following Swimsuit Lean for 30 days, you'll increase your calories from these foods.

# Calorie Ranges for Women

To shed excess body fat on the Swimsuit Lean program, women should allow themselves a minimum of 1500 calories a day and continue to climb to a maximum of 1800 calories a day (see meal plans). That's an increase of 100 calories each week. Start at 1500 calories the first week, and work your way up to 1800 calories the last week of the 30-day period to sustain an encouraging rate of fat loss.

The menu plans in Chapter 12 show you how to do this. If you work out as recommended, exercising will increase the speed of your weekly fat loss. To make sure you're eating enough calories

**WES (At Start, 30 Days)**

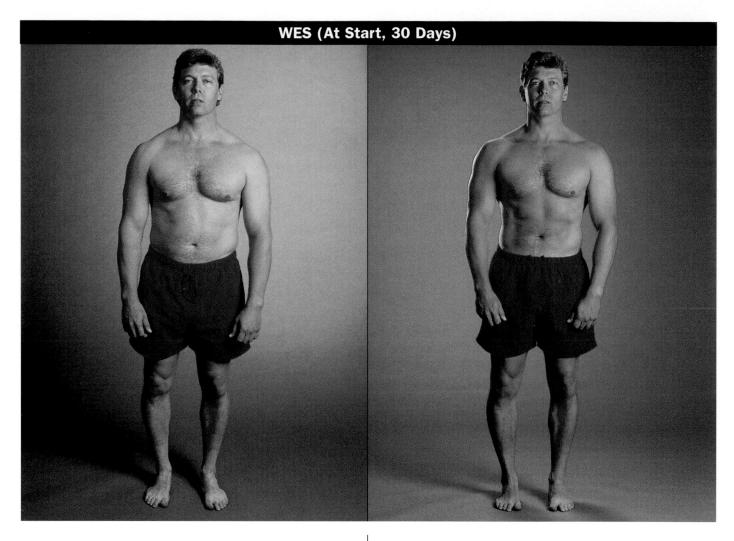

for your activity level, see the optimum fueling formulas that follow.

# Calorie Ranges for Men

Men can handle a greater daily calorie intake than women, so they can start out with higher calories and add more calories on a weekly basis. A man should set his caloric starting point at 2100 the first week, and add 200 calories each week, until reaching 2700 calories or more by the last week of the 30-day program. The menu plans in Chapter 11 illustrate how to make these caloric adjustments. Exercising as recommended will accelerate fat loss. To make sure you're eating enough calo-

ries for your activity level, see the optimum fueling formulas that follow.

# Toward Your Optimum Calories

As you begin the Swimsuit Lean program, you should figure out your optimum caloric goal: the amount of calories you should build toward, based on your sex and activity level. Here's a formula you can use to calculate the number of calories you'll ultimately need each day for optimum fueling and maintenance as your metabolism becomes faster:

# Optimum Fueling Formula

BW . . . . . . . . . . . . . . . . . . . . . . . . . . . . . . . . . . . . . . . . . . . . . . . **Body Weight**
BMR . . . . . . . . . . . . . . . . . . . . . . . . . . . . . . . . . . . . . . . . **Basal Metabolic Rate**
　　　　　　　(the rate at which calories are burned to fuel the body's basic biological function
VMA . . . . . . . . . . . . . . . . . . . . . . . . . . . . . . . **Voluntary Muscular Activity**
SDA . . . . . . . . . . . . . . . . . . . . . . . . . . . . . . . . . . . **Specific Dynamic Action**

**BW/2.2 = BW (\*kg) x .9 (for women) = Women's BW kg**

▼

**BW kg x 24 hrs = BMR**

▼

**BMR x .8 (\*\*This number can vary depending on your activity level) = VMA**

▼

**BMR + VMA = Calories x .1 = SDA**

▼

**BMR + VMA + SDA = Calories for Optimal Fueling**

\* A kilogram (kg) equals 2.2 pounds
\*\* If you are sedentary, use .50 here; moderately active (you exercise three to four times a week, doing aerobics), .65; and very active, .80 (performing the Lean Bodies Workout as described).

To show you how this formula works, let's suppose you're a very active women, weighing 57 kg (or 125 pounds). Your calculation would look like this:

**125 lbs/2.2 = 57 (kg) x .9 (for women) = Women's 51.3 kg**

**51.3 kg x 24 hrs. = 1231. 2 (BMR)**

▼

**1231.2 (BMR) x .8 = 984.96 (VMA)**

▼

**1231.2 (BMR) + 984.96 (VMA) = 2216.16 (Calories) x .1 = 221.6 (SDA)**

▼

**1231.2 (BMR) + 984.96 (VMA) + 221.6 (SDA) = 2437.76 Calories for Optimal Fueling**

Here's a calculation for a very active man who weighs 79 kg (or 175 pounds).

79 kg x 24 hrs. = 1896 (BMR)

▼

1896 (BMR) x .8 = 1516.8 (VMA)

▼

1896 (BMR) + 1516.8 (VMA) = 3412.8 (Calories) x .1 = 341 (SDA)

▼

**1896 (BMR) + 1516.8 (VMA) + 341 (SDA) = 3754 Calories for Optimal Fueling**

**General formula**—For even more precise measurement, have your body composition analyzed, and use your lean mass weight plus ten pounds for your ideal projected weight in the above formula.

# Chapter 6
## *Five Meals a Day*

An interesting phenomenon occurs after you eat a meal: Your body heats up a little bit. This heat is a result of the intense metabolic action involved in digesting and absorbing the food you've eaten. Your metabolic rate actually rises as a result of eating. This elevation in metabolism is technically known as "thermogenesis." It can last for as long as three to four hours after a meal, even longer if the meal includes some protein.

How can you put this scientific fact to work to burn fat? By eating more meals throughout the day!

While following the Swimsuit Lean program, you eat five meals a day—breakfast, lunch, and dinner, plus a mid-morning meal and a mid-afternoon meal. Eating five meals daily, each with some protein, has a stimulating effect on your metabolism. That's just what you need to keep your body's fat-burning wheels in motion.

Here's how to structure your meals for best results. Each main Swimsuit Lean meal is made up of:

❶ **A lean protein**
❷ **One or two starchy carbohydrates**
❸ **One or two lean, fibrous vegetables**

I call the mid-morning and mid-afternoon meals "mini" or "mock" meals. These must be included in your daily menu as well. A mini-meal is approximately one to two ounces of lean protein or low-fat dairy product with 3/4 cup of a starchy carbohydrate. For example:

**❶ A lean protein or low-fat dairy product** (skim milk or non-fat, sugar-free yogurt)

**❷ A starchy carbohydrate**

Mock meals are a convenient way to get in your mid-morning and mid-afternoon meals—perfect for an on-the-go lifestyle. They consist of certain supplements mixed into a delicious shake such as a powdered protein/carbohydrate supplement, mixed with water, Crystal Light, or sugar-free Tang. A sports nutrition bar makes a great mock meal too. Either of these supplements can be eaten along with a starchy carbohydrate, if you wish.

Eating five meals a day really isn't so unusual. Most people do it all the time with between-meal snacks. The problem is, they eat the wrong kinds of foods—foods that are converted easily into body fat. Happily, the foods you're eating on Swimsuit Lean do not do that. They're put to good use in building your body and elevating your metabolism. This all adds up to easier, more effective fat loss.

A word of advice: Please don't skip breakfast. Breakfast is truly the most important meal of the day. Skipping it leads to food cravings later on, intense hunger, and low energy. What's more, studies have found that people who regularly eat breakfast tend to be lean; people who don't tend to be heavy.[1]

The Swimsuit Lean breakfasts include complex carbohydrates to provide energy, fiber to fill you up, and protein to help nutrients release more slowly for even energy levels throughout the morning. If you're not in the habit of eating breakfast, force-feed yourself to do so! Don't be afraid to pack in plenty of calories at breakfast; you have all day to burn them off. Eventually you'll get used to a big breakfast—and even look forward to it.

The menu plans in Chapter 12 show you how the five-meal-a-day structure works. There's no guesswork or room for error if you follow these plans exactly as written.

# Chapter 7
## No More Hunger Pangs

One of the major problems with most restrictive diets is that you feel hungry all the time—so hungry you feel like stuffing yourself. And so off the diet you go, bingeing on high-fat, sugary food and gaining more body fat than you started with. This is certainly a vicious cycle.

I assure you that you won't feel hungry on the Swimsuit Lean program—for several reasons. First, you're eating five times a day, and this includes breakfast, lunch, and dinner, plus two smaller meals at mid-morning and mid-afternoon. On average, you're fueling yourself every three hours.

Generally, the body sends out hunger signals about every four hours by creating hunger pangs and physical sensations such as weakness and shortened attention span. With your Swimsuit Lean eating schedule, you're cutting the body's hunger signals off at the pass. There's no way you can get hungry when eating every three hours!

Stephanie M., a confessed food-lover, agrees: "Eating every few hours is perfect, especially if you like to eat. I'm never hungry. Plus, the program gives me more food choices than I thought I had."

Second, the type of food and the combinations eaten are guaranteed to keep hunger pangs at bay. There's a scientific explanation behind this.

One of the purposes of digestion is to reduce food into smaller units that the body can absorb from the bloodstream. Proteins are broken down into amino acids, carbohydrates into blood sugar (glucose), and fats into fatty acids. Of these, blood sugar has the biggest effect on hunger. When blood sugar levels dip below what the body

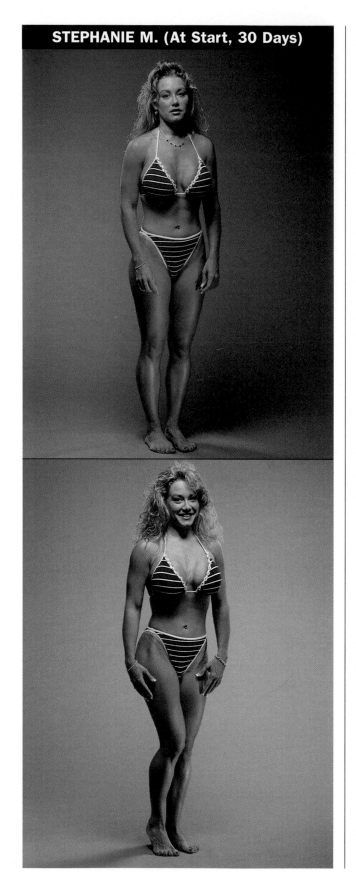

**STEPHANIE M. (At Start, 30 Days)**

needs, signals are sent out and interpreted by the brain as hunger. Conversely, when blood sugar levels are normal, you don't feel hungry; when they're low, you do. You'll also crave sweets.

Certain carbohydrates, namely simple sugars and refined carbohydrates, are converted into blood sugar much more rapidly than natural, starchy, or high-fiber carbohydrates are. This fast conversion results in huge blood sugar spikes. When this happens, the pancreas secretes a large amount of the hormone insulin to normalize blood sugar levels. But after an hour or two, the excess quantity of insulin in the system tends to suppress blood sugar levels—not back to normal but to lower-than-normal levels. The result is hunger pangs and low energy.

On the Swimsuit Lean program, you're eating high-fiber, natural carbohydrates (which tend to convert more slowly into blood sugar) along with lean proteins, a slowly digested food. Together, these foods assist in a slow release of energy, subdue the rate at which carbohydrates are reduced to blood sugar, and minimize the production of insulin. What's more, Swimsuit Lean meals make you feel satisfyingly full, but not too full. Consequently, you do not get hungry later on, and your energy levels are more sustained throughout the day.

Next, there's the issue of exercise—whether or not it makes you feel more hungry and thus causes you to gorge on too much food. Let me set the record straight: Exercise does not make you hungrier, nor does it increase your appetite (your desire for food).

In two recent scientific experiments, it was found that the harder you exercise, the less you want to eat afterwards. Not only that, intense exercise actually suppresses your appetite for a brief period following the workout.[1]

So when you add exercise to your fat-loss efforts, it won't make you hungrier. It will just help you lose more body fat and become more physically fit.

# Chapter 8

## Fluids—What to Drink, What Not to Drink

On the Swimsuit Lean program you're advised to drink plenty of water—between eight to ten large glasses a day. Water is not only the most abundant nutrient in your body (roughly two-thirds of your weight), it is also the most critical. Why? Because it is involved in nearly every process that goes on in your body, from digestion to circulation to excretion. Water, along with other internal fluids, supplies nutrients to nourish body cells and tissues and remove waste products from the body. Water also helps maintain normal body temperature. The many functions of water in the body are summarized in Table 8-1.

Water is important from a fat-burning perspective as well. The kidneys need ample water to do their job of filtering waste products from the body. If water is in short supply, the kidneys can't filter properly, so they turn to the liver for help. One of the liver's many responsibilities is mobilizing stored fat for energy. But when it takes over for the kidneys, the liver can't do its fat-burning job as well. This can hinder fat loss.

The amount of water you need daily depends on your weight. Generally, an an average adult needs a little more than two quarts of water a day to maintain a healthy water balance.[1]

There's an easy way to tell whether or not you've had enough water: Check the color of your urine. Clear-colored urine indicates that you are well-hydrated; dark-colored urine means you are dehydrated. The

| TABLE 8-1 |
|:---:|
| *Functions of Water in the Body* |
| Provides the fluid in which life-sustaining chemical reactions can take place |
| Involved in energy-producing processes |
| Carries nutrients to cells and transports waste products away |
| Serves as a solvent for vitamins, minerals, amino acids, glucose, and other nutrients |
| Regulates body temperature by collecting heat generated by metabolism |
| Facilitates muscular movement through chemical reactions involving nerve transmission |
| Prevents heat cramps and heat exhaustion, two problems caused by water deficiency in the body |

reason for the dark color is an accumulation of metabolic waste not adequately filtered.[2]

Try to drink water throughout the day. Because you'll be exercising on the Swimsuit Lean program, a good rule of thumb to follow is: Drink a glass or two before you exercise, sip water during exercise, and then have another glass or two after exercise.

If you perspire heavily during exercise, weigh yourself before and after your workout. A pound of sweat equals two cups of water—the amount of fluid you should replace. Suppose you drop a pound following a class of intense aerobic dancing. Accordingly, you should re-tank yourself with two cups of water.[3]

There are many types of water you can drink, some more beneficial than others. Most ordinary tap water comes from rivers, streams, and lakes. Unfortunately, it may be contaminated with pollutants, chemicals, and agricultural or industrial wastes. Many of these substances may be carcinogenic, or cancer-inducing, when consumed in large amounts. To be on the safe side, drink bottled spring water or water from the tap that has been purified by a special filtering system. I don't recommend distilled water. Though purified, distilled water is not a good choice because all its minerals are removed during vaporization and condensation. There are other fluids you can drink too, but some you should avoid. Please read the following important instructions about fluids while you're following the Swimsuit Lean program.

# Coffee and Tea

Coffee and other caffeinated beverages are a mixed bag when it comes to health and nutrition. On one hand, caffeine, the active substance in coffee and tea, may cause vitamins and minerals to be flushed out of the body before they can be used, create certain vitamin B deficiencies, and prevent iron from being properly absorbed. Too much caffeine causes the jitters, irritates the stomach lining, and contributes to heartbeat irregularities. Caffeine is also a diuretic, meaning that it promotes water loss from the body.

On the positive side, some research suggests that caffeine may extend performance during exercise—in other words, allow you to work out longer and harder. One reason may be that caffeine increases the level of fatty acids in the blood. When this happens, more fuel (in the form of fatty acids) is available for use by the working muscles.[4] Most of the research in this area, however, has been conducted with athletes. More studies are needed to see what effect, if any, caffeine has on regular exercisers and less active people.

Coffee and other caffeinated drinks can give you a false sense of energy. This occurs because caffeine acts like a sharp poker to spark the adrenal glands. The adrenals release adrenaline, a hormone that allows the body to form energy very quickly in fight-or-flight situations.

Depending on strength, tea contains much less caffeine than coffee and may be a better choice. In the spotlight now is green tea, being widely touted for its many health properties. Green tea is loaded with natural chemicals called flavonoids that may help prevent cancer and reduce cholesterol, among other benefits. Each cup of green tea has about 12 milligrams of caffeine, whereas the more common black tea has between 20 and 110, depending on the brand.[5]

As an alternative to coffee, you may want to make the switch to green tea for its possible nutritive value, or try herbal tea or decaffeinated beverages. Drinking a few cups of coffee or tea does not replace the water you need for the day, however. You still must drink eight to ten glasses daily of pure spring or purified water.

If coffee and tea don't bother you, then you shouldn't have to worry about their potential ill effects. Simply drink them in moderation.

## Diet Soft Drinks

Drinking calorie-free carbonated soft drinks is allowed on the Swimsuit Lean program, but in moderation. These soft drinks contain artificial sweeteners and other chemicals. How they are used by the body is unclear. What's more, soft drinks may decrease calcium levels in the blood, and this action could deplete mineral stores in the bones.

People like diet soft drinks for the caffeine they contain. As noted above, caffeine produces a false sense of energy by stimulating the adrenals.

Diet soft drinks can be counterproductive in another way too. Many people count these beverages as their daily fluid intake and drink them in place of water. As a colleague of mine, Dr. Ron Overberg, puts it: "Would you wash your clothes in diet soda? Then why would you wash your body with it?"

As with other beverages, moderation is the key when including diet soft drinks in your daily menu.

## Fruit Juices

With the exception of tomato or vegetable juice, fruit juices are limited in the initial 30 days on the Swimsuit Lean program. This may sound unusual to you. The reason is that fruit juices can be culprits in promoting body fat—even though they are very nutritious, full of vitamins and minerals. As I explained in Chapter 3, fruit juices are high in a simple sugar called fructose. Because of its chemical make-up and the way it is metabolized, fructose is easily converted into body fat if not used to supply energy.

Let me be perfectly clear: Fruit juice, like fruit, is very healthy. But if you have too much body fat, or have a slow metabolism, you may want to limit fruit juice in the first few weeks to speed your progress in losing body fat.

## Sports Drinks

Sports drinks, also known as fluid-electrolyte beverages, are great for hard-training athletes (especially in hot weather) or for active people who have managed to control their weight and maintain a low body-fat percentage. Under certain exercise conditions, sports drinks help athletes and exercisers replace fluids and essential minerals that are lost in sweat.

But it may be a good idea to pass them up while following the Swimsuit Lean program. One reason is that sports drinks contain simple sugars, which can promote fat storage and thus keep you from getting lean.

# Alcohol

Wine, when taken in moderation (one to two standard-sized drinks a day), has certain beneficial effects on the heart. Also, there are many beneficial enzymes in wine that may aid in digestion.

But as far as fat loss is concerned, it's best to exercise good judgment with regard to alcohol while following the Swimsuit Lean program. Drinking alcohol can actually interfere with your fat-loss efforts. Although a carbohydrate, alcohol is not first converted to glycogen as other carbohydrates are. It is converted instead to fatty acids. What is not used for energy is turned into body fat and stored. Also, when alcohol is in the system, the liver spends a lot of time metabolizing it and can't turn its attention toward burning fat. Some experts have estimated that drinking alcohol cuts your fat-burning potential by as much as one-third.[6]

Alcohol also interferes with the use of carbohydrates during exercise, particularly during prolonged periods of aerobic exercise. This can lead to impaired exercise performance. What's more, alcohol can have a dehydrating effect on the body and blocks the absorption of B-vitamins, which are necessary for energy production.

My advice is to limit alcohol during the initial 30 days of the Swimsuit Lean program. Remember, moderation is the key.

# A Note about Fluid Retention

Period bouts of fluid retention, medically known as edema, can keep you from looking swimsuit lean even after you've shed significant amounts of body fat. Water "dams up" in certain places such as the legs, around the eyelids, even the abdominal area. You look fat even though it's just water weight.

This bloated condition may be the result of any number of factors: excess sodium in the diet, food allergies, hormone imbalances, a hot climate, and diseases such as kidney or heart trouble.

In cases where medical problems for fluid retention have been ruled out, there are some natural, safe precautions you can take to make sure excess water weight doesn't blur the lines of your swimsuit-lean physique. Here are several recommendations:

**❶ Drink plenty of water throughout the day.**
Paradoxically, water is one of the best preventive measures against fluid retention. Your kidneys need a constant supply of water to properly eliminate fluids and waste products from your body. If water is in short supply, the kidneys tend to hoard water, and bloat can set in. Try to drink between eight and ten glasses of pure water daily.

**❷ Moderate your sodium intake.**
Excessive salt also makes your body retain too much water. Lightly salt your food, and try to use less than half a teaspoon when fixing your meals. If you miss the taste of salt on your foods, try a salt substitute or experiment with various herbs and spices in your cooking. The amount of salt the body can handle varies from person to person.

**③ Plan your meals with vegetables that are naturally diuretic.**

Some foods are thought to be diuretic, meaning they help the body eliminate water. These include cucumbers, parsley, watercress, asparagus, and beets. You might try including these on your diet if you suffer from fluid retention.[7]

**④ Supplement your diet with minerals.**

Certain nutrients assist the body in regulating water and are referred to as electrolytes. Sodium, calcium, and chloride are the main electrolytes in the fluid outside cells; potassium, magnesium, and phosphorous are found inside cellular fluid. Electrolytes provide a life-sustaining environment for cells and must be kept in constant balance for good health. These nutrients are lost through perspiration, so active people often have higher requirements. A mineral supplement should always be taken with meals—and only after consulting your physician.

**⑤ Stick to your aerobic exercise program.**

If blood vessels lack resiliency, extra water can flow from them and collect in the tissues, causing water retention. One way to prevent this condition is to exercise aerobically. Aerobic exercise such as walking, jogging, and bicycling improves the resiliency and tone of blood vessels.[8]

# Chapter 9
## Eating Out on Swimsuit Lean

*I* don't expect you to be a hermit while following the Swimsuit Lean program. You are free to go out to restaurants, even fast-food establishments, to enjoy a breakfast, lunch, or dinner out with your friends, family, or business acquaintances. Nor should you pass up invitations to parties or other social events just because you're on a special eating program. One of the many advantages of Swimsuit Lean is its adaptability to any eating-out situation. The foods on this program are served practically everywhere. Keep two simple guidelines in mind:

❶ **Stick to natural foods**—vegetables, whole grains, and lean proteins.
❷ **Order foods cooked without oil, margarine, or butter.**

Most restaurants have the foods you'll be eating while on Swimsuit Lean. The trick is to make sure they're prepared without any fat. Nor should foods be smothered in high-fat sauces. It's critical to stay low-fat throughout the 30-day period. Excess dietary fat is a roadblock to becoming swimsuit lean. Very little energy is required to metabolize fat, compared to other foods. The body simply doesn't work very hard to break down fat, preferring instead to hang onto it rather than burn it for energy. This unmetabolized fat tends to be stored as body fat. The more fat you eat, the more fat you store.

As Lean Body Judy P. says, "I travel for a living as a sales rep. Almost all my meals are eaten out. Even so, I can still follow the Swimsuit Lean eating plan with just a little extra effort."

The following suggestions will help you make the right selections wherever you go:

## HOTEL RESTAURANTS FOR BREAKFAST

■ Order an egg white omelet, cooked with green peppers, onions, and mushrooms, if possible. Be sure that the omelet is cooked without added oil.

■ Order oatmeal, grits, oat bran, or other whole grain cereal with skim milk on the side.

■ Stick to low-sugar fruits such as berries.

■ Drink water.

## ASIAN RESTAURANTS

■ Select entrees made with lean proteins (such as chicken and fish) and vegetables.

■ Order sauce on the side.

■ Request that your rice be steamed.

■ Order your food without the flavor enhancer MSG (this causes allergic reactions in some people, resulting in water retention).

■ Order water or iced tea with lemon.

## MEXICAN RESTAURANTS

■ Rather than snack on a bowl full of fat-laden tortilla chips, ask your server to bring you some corn tortillas to dip.

■ Order fajitas but request that the chicken and vegetables be grilled dry.

■ Grilled chicken, shrimp, or swordfish are always safe.

■ Ask for pico de gallo (a mixture of chopped tomatoes, green peppers, and onions) instead of salsa.

■ If you order rice, be sure that it is steamed.

■ A dinner salad with non-fat salad dressing makes a nice accompaniment to a Mexican meal.

■ Ask for corn tortillas, rather than the flour variety.

■ Avoid corn chips.

■ Order water or iced tea with lemon.

## STEAKHOUSE

■ Order grilled chicken, salmon, or other fish (prepared without oil).

■ As a side dish, select a steamed vegetable such as broccoli, a baked potato, or steamed rice.

■ At the salad bar, stick to fresh vegetables and non-fat salad dressing.

■ Order water or iced tea with lemon.

## HOMESTYLE RESTAURANT

■ For protein, order grilled or lemon chicken or turkey breast.

■ Order steamed rice, a dry baked potato, or corn prepared without butter or margarine.

■ Select steamed vegetables (no sauce or butter), salad with non-fat dressing, or carrot/vegetable medley prepared without butter or margarine.

- Order water or iced tea with lemon.

## DELICATESSEN

- A good protein choice is sliced turkey breast, although make sure it is not smoked. The smoking process uses a lot of oil and salt and may add carcinogenic nitrates to the meat.
- Order steamed vegetable side dishes, if available, or a plain salad (bring your own non-fat dressing).
- Experiment with different mustards to use on your protein and salad selections, rather than mayonnaise or salad dressing.
- Order water or iced tea with lemon.

## FAST FOOD RESTAURANTS

- Limit fast food meals to no more than once a week.
- Select a grilled chicken sandwich (no sauce or mayonnaise and remove bun); baked white fish; or rotisserie chicken (white meat only, with skin removed and meat patted dry). Ask for extra mustard.
- Grilled chicken salads with non-fat salad dressing are a safe bet.
- At the salad bar, stick to fresh vegetables and low-fat or non-fat salad dressing.
- Baked potato and steamed rice (where available) make good starchy carbohydrate choices.
- Order iced water.

## ENTERTAINMENT/SPORTS EVENTS

- Popcorn—as long as it's air-popped—is a good choice.
- Pack a sports nutrition bar for the movies instead of indulging in movie candy.
- A grilled chicken sandwich is fine—but not the bun; it's a refined carbohydrate.
- Non-fat, sugar-free frozen yogurt is safe, but don't eat more than one cup.

## PARTIES

- Eat a meal, or a mock or mini-meal before you go to the party to stave off hunger pangs and cravings.
- Snack on fresh vegetables (but pass up the dip), popcorn (if it's air-popped), or baked tortilla corn chips (just a few).
- Instead of a cocktail, drink a diet soda or carbonated water with a twist of lemon or lime.

## TRAVEL

- Pack sports bars, cut-up fresh vegetables, and cans of water-packed tuna to eat on the road or while in flight.
- Pack rice cakes and baggies of rolled oats (in case there's a microwave in your hotel room).
- In airports, look for popcorn (air-popped, of course), or non-fat, sugar-free frozen yogurt as snack foods.

■ Drink plenty of water if you're flying, since air travel can be quite dehydrating due to cabin pressure and altitude. Avoid caffeine on the flight since it increases fluid loss and may cause dehydration.

When dining out or attending social events, don't worry if servers or hosts give you a funny look. It's your body. Fuel it properly. As I tell people in my Lean Bodies classes: "Be aggressive, but not obsessive."

# Chapter 10
## Swimsuit Lean Guidelines

ere are the key guidelines to follow in order to lose body fat effectively on the Swimsuit Lean program:

1. **Start at the recommended total daily calorie intake**—1500 calories a day for women; 2100 calories a day for men. Each week, add calories. Women should add 100 calories weekly; men, 200. Read Chapter 5 for information on the importance of gradually increasing calories.

2. **To plan your daily menus**, consult the meal planning guidelines in Chapters 11 and 12. With Swimsuit Lean, meal options are already written down for you, but you can adapt them by exchanging various foods with selections from the food list.

3. **Write down what you are going to eat each day.** Creating a food diary like this helps you stick to the program and keep from eating foods that can sabotage your fat-loss efforts. (See The Personal Menu Planner on page 165.)

4. **Do not skip any meals.**

5. **Try not to eat anything two and a half hours before bedtime.** Get all of your calories in by that time. If your schedule does not permit this, make sure your last meal is two and a half hours before bedtime.

6. **Spread your meals throughout the day.** Every time you eat a meal, your metabolism is elevated.

7. **Buy and cook in bulk.** Set aside a morning, an afternoon, or an evening to cook large quantities of food. Store that food in the refrigerator or freezer. That way, you can simply re-heat it or microwave it at meal time.

⑧ Apart from coffee, tea, and diet soft drinks, **drink eight to ten glasses a day of pure water**.

⑨ **All proteins should be very lean.** Remove any skin or visible fat from chicken and turkey before cooking.

⑩ **Eat vegetables without butter, margarine, or sauces.** Experiment with various spices or non-fat butter seasonings on your vegetables. Baked potatoes taste buttery with a teaspoon or two of MCT oil drizzled over them.

⑪ **Consult the *Lean Bodies Cookbook*** (available in paperback) for a variety of delicious ways to prepare your foods.

⑫ You may **use non-fat salad dressings** on salads.

⑬ **Eat mostly the recommended low-sugar fruits** (see Chapter 3) during the 30-day period; other fruits may be added back to your eating program after you begin the Swimsuit Lean maintenance program.

⑭ **Follow the recommended suggestions** for exercise frequency, duration, and intensity as explained in Chapter 15. Doing so will accelerate your fat loss. Additional information on exercise and fat loss can be found in my book, *Lean Bodies Total Fitness*.

## An Important Note about HEALTH STATUS

It is always a wise idea to get your doctor's permission before embarking on any eating or exercise program. If you are currently overweight, you could have health problems that have gone undetected. If you have been somewhat inactive up to now, you should definitely consult a doctor about starting an exercise program and perhaps have a treadmill stress test to verify your present fitness level.

Fortunately, the low-fat, high-fiber natural foods used on the Swimsuit Lean program have been shown to improve nutritional status, just as proper exercise has been shown to improve fitness and vitality. The benefit of the Swimsuit Lean program is to protect you from health problems and help get you into peak shape.

# II

# Swimsuit Lean Meal Plans

# Chapter 11
## Sample Daily Menus

The meal plans that follow provide between 1500 and 2700 calories a day and are appropriate for men and women. Women should start at the 1500-calorie level and add 100 calories each week; men, at the 2100-calorie level, adding 200 calories each week.

Many Americans are in the habit of skipping meals. If you're trying to lose body fat, skipping meals will work against you. Any time you skip a meal, you're setting yourself up for a "hunger surge" in which you might start craving the wrong foods. Follow the menus as written, and you'll be pleasantly surprised by your fat loss and energy levels.

## Burn More Fat
### by Eliminating Starchy Carbohydrates from Your Evening Meal

Reducing the starchy carbohydrates by cutting them in half a few evening meals each week will stimulate your fat-burning power. The elimination or reduction of these carbohydrates makes your body glycogen-needy the next day. Consequently, your body will tap into fatty acids for energy more readily, especially if you do pre-breakfast aerobics (see Chapter 12 for more information). You'll get leaner, faster.

Some people on this program feel a little hungry at night when they've reduced—or cut out—their starchy carbohydrates at the evening meal. **To counteract this, eat an additional serving of lean fibrous vegetables at dinner, along with a little extra protein.**

# 1500-Calorie Meal Plan
## *Week 1*

| BREAKFAST | | |
| --- | --- | --- |
| **LEAN PROTEIN OPTIONS** | **STARCHY CARBOHYDRATE OPTIONS** | **BREAKFAST BLENDS** |
| 4 scrambled egg whites | 2/3 cup raw oats, | 2/3 cup raw oats |
| **or** | **or** | **plus** |
| 10 oz. skim milk | 8 oz. potato or sweet potato, | one of the following proteins: |
| **or** | **or** | 8 oz. yogurt (fat-free, sugar-free) |
| 8 oz yogurt (fat-free, sugar-free) | 2 cups natural whole grain cereal | **or** |
| **or** | (or 200 calories), | 10 oz. skim milk |
| 3 oz. chicken or turkey (white | **or** | **or** |
| meat), fish, or Longhorn beef | 1 1/4 cups shredded wheat | 2 oz. protein powder. Add water and |
| **or** | **or** | ice cubes; blend thoroughly. |
| 1 oz. protein powder mixed with | 1/2 cup grits | Makes a quick, complete Swimsuit |
| water | | Lean breakfast.* |

| MID-MORNING/MID-AFTERNOON | |
| --- | --- |
| **MOCK MEAL OR** | **MINI MEAL** |
| 1 scoop each of protein and carbohydrate powder | A combination of: |
| **or** | 2-3 oz. of lean protein (white meat chicken or turkey, |
| a sports nutrition bar | fish, Longhorn beef, or shrimp; **or** 1 cup skim milk; **or** |
| | 8 oz. yogurt, or 3-6 scrambled egg whites) |
| | **and** |
| | carbohydrate (1/2 cup of rice, corn, beans, or peas; **or** 4 |
| | oz. potato or sweet potato; **or** 100 calories of whole |
| | grain cereal) |

| LUNCH AND DINNER | | |
| --- | --- | --- |
| **LEAN PROTEIN OPTIONS** | **STARCHY CARBOHYDRATE OPTIONS** | **FIBROUS CARBOHYDRATE OPTIONS** |
| 4 oz. of lean protein | 1 cup of rice, corn, beans, or peas | 2 cups of broccoli, cauliflower, |
| (white meat chicken or turkey, | **or** | asparagus, green beans, Brussels |
| fish, Longhorn beef, or shrimp) | 8 oz. potato or sweet potato | sprouts, summer squash, cabbage, |
| | | carrots, Chinese vegetables, |
| | | mushrooms, eggplant, onions, |
| | | tomatoes, peppers, or leafy greens |

* You may add 1 cup of high-fiber, low-sugar fruit such as strawberries or raspberries to the Breakfast Blend.

# 1600-Calorie Meal Plan

## Week 2

### BREAKFAST

| LEAN PROTEIN OPTIONS | STARCHY CARBOHYDRATE OPTIONS | BREAKFAST BLENDS |
|---|---|---|
| 4 scrambled egg whites | 1 cup raw oats | 1 cup raw oats |
| or | or | **plus** |
| 10 oz. skim milk | 12 oz. potato or sweet potato | one of the following proteins: |
| or | or | 8 oz. yogurt (fat-free, sugar-free) |
| 8 oz yogurt (fat-free, sugar-free) | 3 cups natural whole grain cereal (or 300 calories) | or |
| or | or | 10 oz. skim milk |
| 3 oz. chicken or turkey (white meat), fish, or Longhorn beef | 1 3/4 cups shredded wheat | or |
| or | or | 2 oz. protein powder. Add water and ice cubes; blend thoroughly. Makes a quick, complete Swimsuit Lean breakfast.* |
| 1 oz. protein powder mixed with water | 2/3 cup grits | |

### MID-MORNING/MID-AFTERNOON

| MOCK MEAL OR | MINI MEAL |
|---|---|
| 1 scoop each of protein and carbohydrate powder | A combination of: |
| or | 2-3 oz. of lean protein (white meat chicken or turkey, fish, Longhorn beef, or shrimp; **or** 1 cup skim milk; **or** 8 oz. yogurt, or 3-6 scrambled egg whites) |
| a sports nutrition bar | **and** |
| | carbohydrate (1/2 cup of rice, corn, beans, or peas; **or** 4 oz. potato or sweet potato; **or** 100 calories of whole grain cereal) |

### LUNCH AND DINNER

| LEAN PROTEIN OPTIONS | STARCHY CARBOHYDRATE OPTIONS | FIBROUS CARBOHYDRATE OPTIONS |
|---|---|---|
| 4 oz. of lean protein (white meat chicken or turkey, fish, Longhorn beef, or shrimp). | 1 cup of rice, corn, beans, or peas; | 2 cups of broccoli, cauliflower, asparagus, green beans, Brussels sprouts, summer squash, cabbage, carrots, Chinese vegetables, mushrooms, eggplant, onions, tomatoes, peppers, or leafy greens |
| | or | |
| | 8 oz. potato or sweet potato | |

* You may add 1 cup of high-fiber, low-sugar fruit such as strawberries or raspberries to the Breakfast Blend.

# 1700-Calorie Meal Plan
## *Week 3*

| BREAKFAST | | |
|---|---|---|
| **LEAN PROTEIN OPTIONS** | **STARCHY CARBOHYDRATE OPTIONS** | **BREAKFAST BLENDS** |
| 4 scrambled egg whites<br>**or**<br>10 oz. skim milk<br>**or**<br>8 oz yogurt (fat-free, sugar-free)<br>**or**<br>3 oz. chicken or turkey (white meat), fish, or Longhorn beef<br>**or**<br>1 oz. protein powder mixed with water | 1 cup raw oats<br>**or**<br>12 oz. potato or sweet potato<br>**or**<br>3 cups natural whole grain cereal (or 300 calories)<br>**or**<br>1 3/4 cups shredded wheat<br>**or**<br>2/3 cup grits | 1 cup raw oats<br>**plus**<br>one of the following proteins:<br>8 oz. yogurt (fat-free, sugar-free)<br>**or**<br>10 oz. skim milk<br>**or**<br>2 oz. protein powder. Add water and ice cubes; blend thoroughly. Makes a quick, complete Swimsuit Lean breakfast.* |

| MID-MORNING/MID-AFTERNOON | |
|---|---|
| **MOCK MEAL OR** | **MINI MEAL** |
| 1 scoop each of protein and carbohydrate powder<br>**or**<br>a sports nutrition bar | A combination of:<br>2-3 oz. of lean protein (white meat chicken or turkey, fish, Longhorn beef, or shrimp; **or** 1 cup skim milk; **or** 8 oz. yogurt, **or** 3-6 scrambled egg whites)<br>**and**<br>carbohydrate (1 cup of rice, corn, beans, or peas; **or** 8 oz. potato or sweet potato; **or** 200 calories of whole grain cereal) |

| LUNCH AND DINNER | | |
|---|---|---|
| **LEAN PROTEIN OPTIONS** | **STARCHY CARBOHYDRATE OPTIONS** | **FIBROUS CARBOHYDRATE OPTIONS** |
| 4 oz. of lean protein (white meat chicken or turkey, fish, Longhorn beef, or shrimp). | 1 cup of rice, corn, beans, or peas<br>**or**<br>8 oz. potato or sweet potato | 2 cups of broccoli, cauliflower, asparagus, green beans, Brussels sprouts, summer squash, cabbage, carrots, Chinese vegetables, mushrooms, eggplant, onions, tomatoes, peppers, or leafy greens |

* You may add 1 cup of high-fiber, low-sugar fruit such as strawberries or raspberries to the Breakfast Blend.

# 1800-Calorie Meal Plan
## *Week 4*

### BREAKFAST

| LEAN PROTEIN OPTIONS | STARCHY CARBOHYDRATE OPTIONS | BREAKFAST BLENDS |
|---|---|---|
| 4 scrambled egg whites<br><br>**or**<br><br>10 oz. skim milk<br><br>**or**<br><br>8 oz yogurt (fat-free, sugar-free)<br><br>**or**<br><br>3 oz. chicken or turkey (white meat), fish, or Longhorn beef;<br><br>**or**<br><br>1 oz. protein powder mixed with water | 1 cup raw oats<br><br>**or**<br><br>12 oz. potato or sweet potato<br><br>**or**<br><br>3 cups natural whole grain cereal (or 300 calories)<br><br>**or**<br><br>1 3/4 cups shredded wheat<br><br>**or**<br><br>2/3 cup grits | 1 cup raw oats<br><br>**plus**<br><br>one of the following proteins:<br><br>8 oz. yogurt (fat-free, sugar-free)<br><br>**or**<br><br>10 oz. skim milk<br><br>**or**<br><br>2 oz. protein powder. Add water and ice cubes; blend thoroughly. Makes a quick, complete Swimsuit Lean breakfast.* |

### MID-MORNING/MID-AFTERNOON

| MOCK MEAL OR | MINI MEAL |
|---|---|
| 1 scoop each of protein and carbohydrate powder<br><br>**or**<br><br>a sports nutrition bar<br><br>**plus**<br><br>70 calories of lean protein or starchy carbohydrates (approximately 2 oz. of lean protein **or** 1/2 cup starchy carbohydrate) | A combination of:<br><br>2-3 oz. of lean protein (white meat chicken or turkey, fish, Longhorn beef, or shrimp; **or** 1 cup skim milk; **or** 8 oz. yogurt; **or** 3-6 scrambled egg whites)<br><br>**and**<br><br>carbohydrate (1 cup of rice, corn, beans, or peas; **or** 8 oz. potato or sweet potato; **or** 200 calories of whole grain cereal) |

### LUNCH AND DINNER

| LEAN PROTEIN OPTIONS | STARCHY CARBOHYDRATE OPTIONS | FIBROUS CARBOHYDRATE OPTIONS |
|---|---|---|
| 4 oz. of lean protein (white meat chicken or turkey, fish, Longhorn beef, or shrimp) **at lunch**; 7 oz. **at dinner** | 1 cup of rice, corn, beans, or peas<br><br>**or**<br><br>8 oz. potato or sweet potato. | 2 cups of broccoli, cauliflower, asparagus, green beans, Brussels sprouts, summer squash, cabbage, carrots, Chinese vegetables, mushrooms, eggplant, onions, tomatoes, peppers, or leafy greens |

* You may add 1 cup of high-fiber, low-sugar fruit such as strawberries or raspberries to the Breakfast Blend.

# 2100-Calorie Meal Plan
## *Week 1*

| BREAKFAST | | |
|---|---|---|
| **LEAN PROTEIN OPTIONS** | **STARCHY CARBOHYDRATE OPTIONS** | **BREAKFAST BLENDS** |
| 4 scrambled egg whites<br>**or**<br>10 oz. skim milk<br>**or**<br>8 oz yogurt (fat-free, sugar-free)<br>**or**<br>3 oz. chicken or turkey (white meat), fish, or Longhorn beef<br>**or**<br>1 oz. protein powder mixed with water | 1 cup raw oats<br>**or**<br>12 oz. potato or sweet potato<br>**or**<br>3 cups natural whole grain cereal, (or 300 calories)<br>**or**<br>1 3/4 cups shredded wheat<br>**or**<br>2/3 cup grits | 1 cup raw oats<br>**plus**<br>one of the following proteins:<br>8 oz. yogurt (fat-free, sugar-free)<br>**or**<br>10 oz. skim milk<br>**or**<br>2 oz. protein powder. Add water and ice cubes; blend thoroughly. Makes a quick, complete Swimsuit Lean breakfast.* |

| MID-MORNING/MID-AFTERNOON | |
|---|---|
| **MOCK MEAL OR** | **MINI MEAL** |
| 1 scoop each of protein and carbohydrate powder<br>**or**<br>a sports nutrition bar | A combination of:<br>2-3 oz. of lean protein (white meat chicken or turkey, fish, Longhorn beef, or shrimp; **or** 1 cup skim milk; **or** 8 oz. yogurt; **or** 3-6 scrambled egg whites)<br>**and**<br>carbohydrate (1/2 cup of rice, corn, beans, or peas; **or** 8 oz. potato or sweet potato; **or** 100 calories of whole grain cereal) |

| LUNCH AND DINNER | | |
|---|---|---|
| **LEAN PROTEIN OPTIONS** | **STARCHY CARBOHYDRATE OPTIONS** | **FIBROUS CARBOHYDRATE OPTIONS** |
| 6 oz. of lean protein (white meat chicken or turkey, fish, Longhorn beef, or shrimp). | 2 cups of rice, corn, beans, or peas<br>**or**<br>16 oz. potato or sweet potato | 2 cups of broccoli, cauliflower, asparagus, green beans, Brussels sprouts, summer squash, cabbage, carrots, Chinese vegetables, mushrooms, eggplant, onions, tomatoes, peppers, or leafy greens |

* You may add 1 cup of high-fiber, low-sugar fruit such as strawberries or raspberries to the Breakfast Blend.

# 2300-Calorie Meal Plan
## *Week 2*

### BREAKFAST

| LEAN PROTEIN OPTIONS | STARCHY CARBOHYDRATE OPTIONS | BREAKFAST BLENDS |
|---|---|---|
| 4 scrambled egg whites<br><br>or<br><br>10 oz. skim milk<br><br>or<br><br>8 oz yogurt (fat-free, sugar-free)<br><br>or<br><br>3 oz. chicken or turkey (white meat), fish, or Longhorn beef; or 1 oz. protein powder mixed with water | 1 1/3 cups raw oats<br><br>or<br><br>16 oz. potato or sweet potato<br><br>or<br><br>4 cups natural whole grain cereal, (or 400 calories)<br><br>or<br><br>2 2/3 cups shredded wheat<br><br>or<br><br>1 cup grits | 1 1/3 cup raw oats<br><br>plus<br><br>one of the following proteins:<br> 8 oz. yogurt (fat-free, sugar-free)<br><br>or<br><br>10 oz. skim milk<br><br>or<br><br>2 oz. protein powder. Add water and ice cubes; blend thoroughly. Makes a quick, complete Swimsuit Lean breakfast.* |

### MID-MORNING/MID-AFTERNOON

| MOCK MEAL OR | MINI MEAL |
|---|---|
| 1 scoop each of protein and carbohydrate powder<br>or<br>a sports nutrition bar<br>plus<br>70 calories of lean protein or starchy carbohydrates (approximately 2 oz. of lean protein or 1/2 cup starchy carbohydrate) | A combination of:<br>2-3 oz. of lean protein (white meat chicken or turkey, fish, Longhorn beef, or shrimp; or 1 cup skim milk; or 8 oz. yogurt; or 3-6 scrambled egg whites)<br>and<br>carbohydrate (1 cup of rice, corn, beans, or peas; or 8 oz. potato or sweet potato; or 200 calories of whole grain cereal). |

### LUNCH AND DINNER

| LEAN PROTEIN OPTIONS | STARCHY CARBOHYDRATE OPTIONS | FIBROUS CARBOHYDRATE OPTIONS |
|---|---|---|
| 6 oz. of lean protein (white meat chicken or turkey, fish, Longhorn beef, or shrimp) | 2 cups of rice, corn, beans, or peas<br><br>or<br><br>16 oz. potato or sweet potato | 2 cups of broccoli, cauliflower, asparagus, green beans, Brussels sprouts, summer squash, cabbage, carrots, Chinese vegetables, mushrooms, eggplant, onions, tomatoes, peppers, or leafy greens |

* You may add 1 cup of high-fiber, low-sugar fruit such as strawberries or raspberries to the Breakfast Blend.

# 2500-Calorie Meal Plan
## *Week 3*

| BREAKFAST | | |
|---|---|---|
| **LEAN PROTEIN OPTIONS** | **STARCHY CARBOHYDRATE OPTIONS** | **BREAKFAST BLENDS** |
| 4 scrambled egg whites | 1 2/3 cups raw oats | 1 2/3 cup raw oats |
| or | or | **plus** |
| 10 oz. skim milk | 20 oz. potato or sweet potato | one of the following proteins: |
| or | or | 8 oz. yogurt (fat-free, sugar-free0 |
| 8 oz yogurt (fat-free, sugar-free) | 5 cups natural whole grain cereal, (or 500 calories) | or |
| or | or | 10 oz. skim milk |
| 3 oz. chicken or turkey (white meat), fish, or Longhorn beef | 3 cups shredded wheat | or |
| or | or | 2 oz. protein powder. Add water and ice cubes; blend thoroughly. Makes a quick, complete Swimsuit Lean breakfast.* |
| 1 oz. protein powder mixed with water | 1 cup grits | |

| MID-MORNING/MID-AFTERNOON | |
|---|---|
| **MOCK MEAL OR** | **MINI MEAL** |
| 1 scoop each of protein and carbohydrate powder | A combination of: |
| or | 2-3 oz. of lean protein (white meat chicken or turkey, fish, Longhorn beef, or shrimp; **or** 1 cup skim milk; **or** 8 oz. yogurt; **or** 3-6 scrambled egg whites) |
| a sports nutrition bar. | **and** |
| **Add** an extra sports nutrition bar before dinner. | carbohydrate (1 cup of rice, corn, beans, or peas; **or** 8 oz. potato or sweet potato; **or** 200 calories of whole grain cereal) |

| LUNCH AND DINNER | | |
|---|---|---|
| **LEAN PROTEIN OPTIONS** | **STARCHY CARBOHYDRATE OPTIONS** | **FIBROUS CARBOHYDRATE OPTIONS** |
| 6 oz. of lean protein (white meat chicken or turkey, fish, Longhorn beef, or shrimp) | 2 cups of rice, corn, beans, or peas | 2 cups of broccoli, cauliflower, asparagus, green beans, Brussels sprouts, summer squash, cabbage, carrots, Chinese vegetables, mushrooms, eggplant, onions, tomatoes, peppers, or leafy greens |
| | or | |
| | 16 oz. potato or sweet potato | |

* You may add 1 cup of high-fiber, low-sugar fruit such as strawberries or raspberries to the Breakfast Blend.

# 2700-Calorie Meal Plan
## *Week 4*

| BREAKFAST | | |
| --- | --- | --- |
| **LEAN PROTEIN OPTIONS** | **STARCHY CARBOHYDRATE OPTIONS** | **BREAKFAST BLENDS** |
| 4 scrambled egg whites<br>**or**<br>10 oz. skim milk<br>**or**<br>8 oz yogurt (fat-free, sugar-free)<br>3 oz. chicken or turkey (white meat), fish, or Longhorn beef<br>**or**<br>1 oz. protein powder mixed with water | 1 2/3 cups raw oats<br>**or**<br>20 oz. potato or sweet potato<br>**or**<br>5 cups natural whole grain cereal, (or 500 calories)<br>**or**<br>3 cups shredded wheat<br>**or**<br>1 cup grits | 1 2/3 cup raw oats<br>**plus**<br>one of the following proteins:<br>8 oz. yogurt (fat-free, sugar-free)<br>**or**<br>10 oz. skim milk<br>**or**<br>2 oz. protein powder. Add water and ice cubes; blend thoroughly. Makes a quick, complete Swimsuit Lean breakfast.* |

| MID-MORNING/MID-AFTERNOON | |
| --- | --- |
| **MOCK MEAL OR** | **MINI MEAL** |
| 1 scoop each of protein and carbohydrate powder<br>**or**<br>a sports nutrition bar<br>**Add** an extra sports nutrition bar before dinner. | A combination of:<br>2-3 oz. of lean protein (white meat chicken or turkey, fish, Longhorn beef, or shrimp; **or** 1 cup skim milk; **or** 8 oz. yogurt; **or** 3-6 scrambled egg whites)<br>**and**<br>carbohydrate (1 cup of rice, corn, beans, or peas; **or** 8 oz. potato or sweet potato; **or** 200 calories of whole grain cereal) |

| LUNCH AND DINNER | | |
| --- | --- | --- |
| **LEAN PROTEIN OPTIONS** | **STARCHY CARBOHYDRATE OPTIONS** | **FIBROUS CARBOHYDRATE OPTIONS** |
| 8 oz. of lean protein (white meat chicken or turkey, fish, Longhorn beef, or shrimp) | 2 cups of rice, corn, beans, or peas;<br>**or**<br>16 oz. potato or sweet potato | 3 cups of broccoli, cauliflower, asparagus, green beans, Brussels sprouts, summer squash, cabbage, carrots, Chinese vegetables, mushrooms, eggplant, onions, tomatoes, peppers, or leafy greens. |

* You may add 1 cup of high-fiber, low-sugar fruit such as strawberries or raspberries to the Breakfast Blend.

# Real-Life Menu Planning

It's easy to turn the above guidelines into your own personalized menu. Here are several examples showing how participants planned their meals, using the Swimsuit Lean menu guidelines. Their menus may give you some additional ideas. Then you can plan your own meals, using the Personal Menu Planner on page 165.

## David W.*

| | | |
|---|---|---|
| **Breakfast** | Protein powder | 2 scoops |
| | Carbohydrate powder | 2 cups |
| | Oatmeal, uncooked | 1 cup |
| | Yogurt | 1/2 cup |
| | Skim milk | 1 cup |
| | Strawberries | 2 scoops |
| **Mini/Mock Meal** | Egg whites | 2 |
| | Baked potato | 4 oz. |
| | Tuna | 6 oz. |
| | Picante sauce | 2 tbsp. |
| | Protein powder | 1 scoop |
| | Carbohydrate powder | 1 scoop |
| **Lunch** | Turkey | 8 oz. |
| | Green salad | 1 cup |
| | Low-fat ranch dressing | 1 tsp. |
| | Pinto beans | 1 1/2 cups |
| | Baked potato | 15 oz. |
| **Mini/Mock Meal** | Sports bar | 1 |
| | Protein powder | 2 scoops |
| | Carbohydrate powder | 1 scoop |
| | Lean Bodies Waffle** | 1 |
| **Dinner** | Blackened cod | 12 oz. |
| | New potatoes | 8 oz. |
| | Corn | 1 cup |

*David ate the most calories of anyone in our initial program—and gained muscle while losing body fat.

** See Lean Bodies Cookbook for recipe.

## Larry K.

| Breakfast | Oatmeal, uncooked | 1 1/2 cups |
|---|---|---|
|  | Egg whites | 4 |
|  | **or:** |  |
|  | Yogurt | 8 oz. |
|  | Oatmeal, uncooked | 1 2/3 cups |
|  | Blueberries | 1/4 cup |
|  | Equal | 2 packets |
| Mini/Mock Meal | Sports nutrition bar | 1 bar |
| Lunch | Chicken or fish | 8 oz. |
|  | Potato or sweet potato | 1 |
|  | Corn or peas | 10 oz. |
|  | Salad with fat-free dressing | 16 oz. |
|  | Green beans, squash, or asparagus | 16 oz. |
| Mini/Mock Meal | Sports nutrition bar | 1 bar |
| Dinner | Virtually the same as lunch. On specific days, I would eliminate starchy carbohydrates at my evening meal, as recommended by the program, and try to add another potato or serving of starchy carbohydrate at lunch, or eat an additional sports nutrition bar. |  |

## Sylvia

| Breakfast | Egg whites | 4 |
|---|---|---|
|  | Oatmeal, uncooked | 1/3 cup |
| Mini/Mock Meal | Sports nutrition bar | 1 |
| Lunch | Chicken | 4 oz. |
|  | Egg whites | 3 |
|  | Corn | 1 cup |
|  | Tomatoes | 2 |
|  | Cucumber | 6 slices |
| Mini/Mock Meal | Tuna | 2.5 oz. |
|  | Peas | 1/2 cup |
| Dinner | Chicken | 4 oz. |
|  | Egg whites | 4 |
|  | Green beans | 1 cup |
|  | Tomatoes | 2 |
|  | Raw cauliflower | 1/2 cup |
|  | Cucumber | 6 slices |
|  | Baby carrots | 4 |

## Jerry M.

| MEAL | FOODS | QUANTITY |
|------|-------|----------|
| **Breakfast** | Egg whites | 5 |
| | Oatmeal, uncooked | 1 cup |
| | Potato | 8 oz. |
| **Mini/Mock Meal** | *Breakfast Blend:* | |
| | Oatmeal, uncooked | 1/2 cup |
| | Yogurt | 8 oz. |
| | Non-fat chocolate powder | 1 scoop |
| **Lunch** | Chicken or tuna | 6 oz. |
| | Vegetables - greens, carrots, celery, and cucumbers | 2 cups |
| | Rice | 1 cup |
| | Beans | 1 cup |
| | Potato | 8 oz. |
| **Mini/Mock Meal** | *Breakfast Blend:* | |
| | Oatmeal, uncooked | 1/2 cup |
| | Yogurt | 8 oz. |
| | Non-fat chocolate powder | 1 scoop |
| **Dinner** | Chicken | 6 oz. |
| | Broccoli | 2 cups |
| | Carrot sticks | 2 large |

### NEED A FAST RECIPE THE FAMILY WILL LOVE?

On a large sheet of foil, place a turkey or chicken breast fillet. Top with onion, chopped potatoes, sliced carrots, and spices to taste (bayleaf or Mrs. Dash are nice), plus a generous dash of lemon juice. Roll up tightly and bake at 350 degrees for approximately 30 minutes. We call this dish *The Hobo Dinner** at our house. (Orange roughy, a mellow-flavored white fish, works well in this recipe too.)

*My thanks to Kathy Coker for this recipe that she provided to our Lean Bodies classes.

# Cooking Tips

Once you have a week of high-energy, lean eating under your belt (which hopefully is smaller), you may be ready for some creativity in your cooking. The *Lean Bodies Cookbook* is your best friend in this regard. But if you don't have a copy yet, consider converting some of your favorite recipes to lean treats. Here are some suggestions:

■ Replace oil or fat in marinades, sauces, and salad dressings with compatible liquids like defatted chicken broth, vegetable broth, lemon juice, lime juice, flavored vinegars, tomato juice, vegetable juice, or lite soy sauce.

■ Experiment with herbs. If you like your foods well-seasoned, try recipes that call for basil, bay leaves, cayenne pepper, chili powder, cumin, dill weed, dry mustard, garlic, oregano, rosemary, sage, or thyme. If you like foods that emphasize sweetness, choose recipes that contain cardamom, cinnamon, curry, ginger, marjoram, mint, or nutmeg.

■ Replace the conventional oil in salad dressing recipes with MCT oil. Any oil and vinegar or French dressing recipe converts beautifully.

## PERSONAL MENU PLANNER

Date:

| MEAL | FOODS | CALORIES |
|------|-------|----------|
| **Breakfast** | | |
| | | |
| | | |
| | | |
| | | |
| **Mini/Mock Meal** | | |
| | | |
| | | |
| | | |
| **Lunch** | | |
| | | |
| | | |
| | | |
| | | |
| **Mini/Mock Meal** | | |
| | | |
| | | |
| | | |
| **Dinner** | | |
| | | |
| | | |
| | | |
| | | |
| | | |

If you wish you may spread your calories over six meals a day instead of five. Just follow the aforementioned meal plans, but split up lunch or dinner to reach a total of six meals.

## PERSONAL MENU PLANNER                                    **Date:**

| MEAL | FOODS | CALORIES |
|---|---|---|
| **Breakfast** | | |
| | | |
| | | |
| | | |
| | | |
| | | |
| **Mini/Mock Meal** | | |
| | | |
| | | |
| **Lunch** | | |
| | | |
| | | |
| | | |
| | | |
| | | |
| | | |
| **Mini/Mock Meal** | | |
| | | |
| | | |
| **Dinner** | | |
| | | |
| | | |
| | | |
| | | |
| | | |
| | | |
| | | |
| | | |

If you wish you may spread your calories over six meals a day instead of five. Just follow the afore-mentioned meal plans, but split up lunch or dinner to reach a total of six meals.

# Chapter 12
## Swimsuit Lean—Day by Day

ere is a day-by-day program that outlines exactly what to do each day while following Swimsuit Lean. For information on how to put together each meal, review the sample daily menus in the previous chapter. This program eliminates any guesswork and should function as your roadmap toward becoming swimsuit lean.

Please note that aerobic exercise is prescribed for certain times of the day—before breakfast and before retiring in the evening. There are important fat-burning reasons for this.

Sleeping through the night is like an all-night fast. When you wake up in the morning, your body is lower on glycogen. But what better time to get moving! Rise and shine with 30 minutes of aerobics—before breakfast. With less glycogen, your body has to get fuel from somewhere, so it starts mobilizing fatty acids from fat stores. What happens theoretically is this: More body fat is burned as a result, and you're quickly on your way to a leaner physique.

There's more: Exercising aerobically first thing in the morning ensures that your metabolism stays cranked up for the rest of the day. Your meals that day are metabolized for energy more efficiently. Plus, the carbohydrates you eat head straight to the glycogen-needy muscles and are less likely to be converted to body fat.

*(Note: If you're a cardiac patient, consult your cardiologist on the suitable time of day for performing aerobics.)*

An additional session of aerobic exercise is recommended in the evenings several times each week. Wait a comfortable time after dinner, then go for a 30-minute run, brisk walk, or other aerobic activity. But afterwards, do not eat any carbohydrates. Get a good night's sleep. The next morning, your body will really be glycogen-needy, thanks to the previous night's exercise. After waking up, do another 30 minutes of aerobics—before breakfast. Your body has no choice but to burn extra fat for fuel.

For complete information on the Swimsuit Lean workout, consult Chapters 13 through 18.

# Key Points:

**1** Your aerobics can be performed before breakfast, after dinner, or immediately following your strength training routine.

**2** You can strength train more times during the week, if you wish.

**3** Strength training can be performed on days other than those shown. Make sure you rest muscle groups at least 48 hours before working them again. The time of day you strength train does not matter, as long you have had a meal at least an hour before you work out.

**4** Gradually increase your calories, week by week, as suggested on the Swimsuit Lean eating program.

**5** If you need to, take a break from aerobics one day a week.

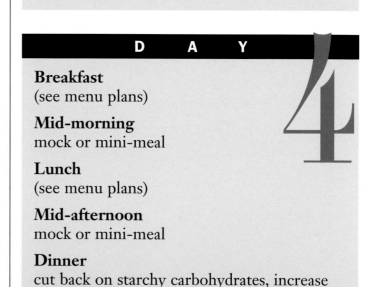

**DAY 1**

**Pre-breakfast aerobics**
30 minutes

**Breakfast**
(see menu plans)

**Mid-morning**
mock or mini-meal

**Lunch**
(see menu plans)

**Mid-afternoon**
mock or mini-meal

**Dinner**
cut back on starchy carbohydrates, increase protein by 1 to 2 oz.; eat up to 2 cups of fibrous vegetables (more if you wish).

**DAY 4**

**Breakfast**
(see menu plans)

**Mid-morning**
mock or mini-meal

**Lunch**
(see menu plans)

**Mid-afternoon**
mock or mini-meal

**Dinner**
cut back on starchy carbohydrates, increase protein by 1 to 2 oz.; eat up to 2 cups of fibrous vegetables (more if you wish).

**Perform your strength training workout today.**

## DAY 2

**Pre-breakfast aerobics**
30 minutes

**Breakfast**
(see menu plans)

**Mid-morning**
mock or mini-meal

**Lunch**
(see menu plans)

**Mid-afternoon**
mock or mini-meal

**Dinner**
(see menu plans; eat a higher protein starchy carbohydrate such as legumes, if you wish)

**Perform your strength training workout today.**

## DAY 3

**Pre-breakfast aerobics**
30 minutes

**Breakfast**
(see menu plans)

**Mid-morning**
mock or mini-meal

**Lunch**
(see menu plans)

**Mid-afternoon**
mock or mini-meal

**Dinner**
cut back on starchy carbohydrates, increase protein by 1 to 2 oz.; eat up to 2 cups of fibrous vegetables (more if you wish).

## DAY 5

**Pre-breakfast aerobics**
30 minutes

**Breakfast**
(see menu plans)

**Mid-morning**
mock or mini-meal

**Lunch**
(see menu plans)

**Mid-afternoon**
mock or mini-meal

**Dinner**
cut back on starchy carbohydrates, increase protein by 1 to 2 oz.; eat up to 2 cups of fibrous vegetables (more if you wish).

## DAY 6

**Pre-breakfast aerobics**
30 minutes

**Breakfast**
(see menu plans)

**Mid-morning**
mock or mini-meal

**Lunch**
(see menu plans)

**Mid-afternoon**
mock or mini-meal

**Dinner**
cut back on starchy carbohydrates, increase protein by 1 to 2 oz.; eat up to 2 cups of fibrous vegetables (more if you wish).

## DAY 7

**Breakfast**
(see menu plans)

**Mid-morning**
mock or mini-meal

**Lunch**
(see menu plans)

**Mid-afternoon**
mock or mini-meal

**Dinner**
cut back on starchy carbohydrates, increase protein by 1 to 2 oz.; eat up to 2 cups of fibrous vegetables (more if you wish).

## DAY 8

**Pre-breakfast aerobics**
30 minutes

**Breakfast**
(see menu plans)

**Mid-morning**
mock or mini-meal

**Lunch**
(see menu plans)

**Mid-afternoon**
mock or mini-meal

**Dinner**
cut back on starchy carbohydrates, increase protein by 1 to 2 oz.; eat up to 2 cups of fibrous vegetables (more if you wish).

## DAY 11

**Breakfast**
(see menu plans)

**Mid-morning**
mock or mini-meal

**Lunch**
(see menu plans)

**Mid-afternoon**
mock or mini-meal

**Dinner**
(see menu plans; eat a higher protein starchy carbohydrate such as legumes, if you wish)

**Perform your strength training workout today.**

## DAY 12

**Pre-breakfast aerobics**
30 minutes

**Breakfast**
(see menu plans)

**Mid-morning**
mock or mini-meal

**Lunch**
(see menu plans)

**Mid-afternoon**
mock or mini-meal

**Dinner**
cut back on starchy carbohydrates, increase protein by 1 to 2 oz.; eat up to 2 cups of fibrous vegetables (more if you wish).

## DAY 9

**Pre-breakfast aerobics**
30 minutes

**Breakfast**
(see menu plans)

**Mid-morning**
mock or mini-meal

**Lunch**
(see menu plans)

**Mid-afternoon**
mock or mini-meal

**Dinner**
(see menu plans; eat a higher protein starchy carbohydrate such as legumes, if you wish)

**Perform your strength training workout today.**

## DAY 10

**Pre-breakfast aerobics**
30 minutes

**Breakfast**
(see menu plans)

**Mid-morning**
mock or mini-meal

**Lunch**
(see menu plans)

**Mid-afternoon**
mock or mini-meal

**Dinner**
cut back on starchy carbohydrates, increase protein by 1 to 2 oz.; eat up to 2 cups of fibrous vegetables (more if you wish).

## DAY 13

**Pre-breakfast aerobics**
40 minutes

**Breakfast**
(see menu plans)

**Mid-morning**
mock or mini-meal

**Lunch**
(see menu plans)

**Mid-afternoon**
mock or mini-meal

**Dinner**
cut back on starchy carbohydrates, increase protein by 1 to 2 oz.; eat up to 2 cups of fibrous vegetables (more if you wish).

## DAY 14

**Breakfast**
(see menu plans)

**Mid-morning**
mock or mini-meal

**Lunch**
(see menu plans)

**Mid-afternoon**
mock or mini-meal

**Dinner**
cut back on starchy carbohydrates, increase protein by 1 to 2 oz.; eat up to 2 cups of fibrous vegetables (more if you wish).

# D A Y 15

**Pre-breakfast aerobics**
40 minutes

**Breakfast**
(see menu plans)

**Mid-morning**
mock or mini-meal

**Lunch**
(see menu plans)

**Mid-afternoon**
mock or mini-meal

**Dinner**
cut back on starchy carbohydrates, increase protein by 1 to 2 oz.; eat up to 2 cups of fibrous vegetables (more if you wish).

**Aerobics**
30 minutes

# D A Y 16

**Pre-breakfast aerobics**
30 minutes

**Breakfast**
(see menu plans)

**Mid-morning**
mock or mini-meal

**Lunch** (see menu plans)

**Mid-afternoon**
mock or mini-meal

**Dinner**
(see menu plans; eat a higher protein starchy carbohydrate such as legumes, if you wish)

**Perform your strength training workout today.**

# D A Y 19

**Pre-breakfast aerobics**
45 minutes

**Breakfast**
(see menu plans)

**Mid-morning**
mock or mini-meal

**Lunch**
(see menu plans)

**Mid-afternoon**
mock or mini-meal

**Dinner**
cut back on starchy carbohydrates, increase protein by 1 to 2 oz.; eat up to 2 cups of fibrous vegetables (more if you wish).

# D A Y 20

**Pre-breakfast aerobics**
45 minutes

**Breakfast**
(see menu plans)

**Mid-morning**
mock or mini-meal

**Lunch**
(see menu plans)

**Mid-afternoon**
mock or mini-meal

**Dinner**
cut back on starchy carbohydrates, increase protein by 1 to 2 oz.; eat up to 2 cups of fibrous vegetables (more if you wish).

## DAY 17

**Pre-breakfast aerobics**
45 minutes

**Breakfast**
(see menu plans)

**Mid-morning**
mock or mini-meal

**Lunch**
(see menu plans)

**Mid-afternoon**
mock or mini-meal

**Dinner**
cut back on starchy carbohydrates, increase protein by 1 to 2 oz.; eat up to 2 cups of fibrous vegetables (more if you wish).

**Aerobics**
30 minutes

## DAY 18

**Breakfast**
(see menu plans)

**Mid-morning**
mock or mini-meal

**Lunch**
(see menu plans)

**Mid-afternoon**
mock or mini-meal

**Dinner**
(see menu plans; eat a higher protein starchy carbohydrate such as legumes, if you wish)

**Perform your strength training workout today.**

**Aerobics**
30 minutes

## DAY 21

**Pre-breakfast aerobics**
45 minutes

**Breakfast**
(see menu plans)

**Mid-morning**
mock or mini-meal

**Lunch**
(see menu plans)

**Mid-afternoon**
mock or mini-meal

**Dinner**
cut back on starchy carbohydrates, increase protein by 1 to 2 oz.; eat up to 2 cups of fibrous vegetables (more if you wish).

## DAY 22

**Pre-breakfast aerobics**
45 minutes

**Breakfast**
(see menu plans)

**Mid-morning**
mock or mini-meal

**Lunch**
(see menu plans)

**Mid-afternoon**
mock or mini-meal

**Dinner**
cut back on starchy carbohydrates, increase protein by 1 to 2 oz.; eat up to 2 cups of fibrous vegetables (more if you wish).

**Aerobics**
30 minutes

## DAY 23

**Aerobics**
30 minutes

**Breakfast**
(see menu plans)

**Mid-morning**
mock or mini-meal

**Lunch** (see menu plans)

**Mid-afternoon**
mock or mini-meal

**Dinner**
(see menu plans; eat a higher protein starchy carbohydrate such as legumes, if you wish)

**Perform your strength training workout today.**

**Aerobics**
30 minutes (at least one aerobic session, the second is optional)

## DAY 24

**Pre-breakfast aerobics**
45 minutes

**Breakfast**
(see menu plans)

**Mid-morning**
mock or mini-meal

**Lunch**
(see menu plans)

**Mid-afternoon**
mock or mini-meal

**Dinner**
cut back on starchy carbohydrates, increase protein by 1 to 2 oz.; eat up to 2 cups of fibrous vegetables (more if you wish).

## DAY 27

**Pre-breakfast aerobics**
45 minutes

**Breakfast**
(see menu plans)

**Mid-morning**
mock or mini-meal

**Lunch**
(see menu plans)

**Mid-afternoon**
mock or mini-meal

**Dinner**
cut back on starchy carbohydrates, increase protein by 1 to 2 oz.; eat up to 2 cups of fibrous vegetables (more if you wish).

**Aerobics**
30 minutes

## DAY 28

**Pre-breakfast aerobics**
45 minutes

**Breakfast**
(see menu plans)

**Mid-morning**
mock or mini-meal

**Lunch**
(see menu plans)

**Mid-afternoon**
mock or mini-meal

**Dinner**
cut back on starchy carbohydrates, increase protein by 1 to 2 oz.; eat up to 2 cups of fibrous vegetables (more if you wish).

## DAY 25

**Aerobics**
45 minutes

**Breakfast**
(see menu plans)

**Mid-morning**
mock or mini-meal

**Lunch**
(see menu plans)

**Mid-afternoon**
mock or mini-meal

**Dinner**
(see menu plans; eat a higher protein starchy carbohydrate such as legumes, if you wish.)

**Perform your strength training workout today.**

## DAY 26

**Pre-breakfast aerobics**
45 minutes

**Breakfast**
(see menu plans)

**Mid-morning**
mock or mini-meal

**Lunch**
(see menu plans)

**Mid-afternoon**
mock or mini-meal

**Dinner**
cut back on starchy carbohydrates, increase protein by 1 to 2 oz.; eat up to 2 cups of fibrous vegetables (more if you wish).

**Aerobics**
30 minutes

## DAY 29

**Pre-breakfast aerobics**
45 minutes

**Breakfast**
(see menu plans)

**Mid-morning**
mock or mini-meal

**Lunch**
(see menu plans)

**Mid-afternoon**
mock or mini-meal

**Dinner**
cut back on starchy carbohydrates, increase protein by 1 to 2 oz.; eat up to 2 cups of fibrous vegetables (more if you wish).

**Aerobics**
30 minutes

## DAY 30

**Pre-breakfast aerobics**
45 minutes

**Breakfast**
(see menu plans)

**Mid-morning**
mock or mini-meal

**Lunch**
(see menu plans)

**Mid-afternoon**
mock or mini-meal

**Dinner**
cut back on starchy carbohydrates, increase protein by 1 to 2 oz.; eat up to 2 cups of fibrous vegetables (more if you wish).

**Aerobics**
30 minutes

# III

# The Swimsuit Lean Workout

# Chapter 13

## *Anti-Fat Exercise*

For fat loss, diet alone just doesn't cut it. In one scientific study, weight loss was evaluated in two groups of women: those who just dieted and those who dieted *and* exercised aerobically. Both groups lost about the same amount of weight, but the composition of their weight loss was different. The exercise group lost a lot more fat, while the diet-only group lost mostly muscle.[1] Similar studies have turned up similar results: When you try to lose fat without exercising, more of your loss will be muscle and less will be fat. Your goal must be twofold: to shed as much fat as possible and to develop additional lean muscle. Exercise can help you do that—in a number of ways.

## Boost Your Metabolism with Exercise

One key to burning more fat is to recharge your metabolism. Exercise can help. When you exercise, your metabolism not only increases but also *stays elevated for a period of time after you exercise*. Scientists call this response "excess post-exercise oxygen consumption," also known as "caloric afterburn."

You can maximize your own caloric afterburn in several ways. One involves the duration, or length, of your exercise session. In one study, five men rode a stationary bicycle at a moderate intensity, randomly varying the length of their rides each day in 30-minute, 45-minute, and 60-minute periods. The researchers found that after the 30-minute ride, the metabolism stayed elevated for 130 minutes; after the 45-minute ride, the metabolism stayed high for 205 minutes. Following the 60-minute ride, the metabolism remained elevated for 455 minutes.[2] So the longer you work out, the greater your caloric afterburn and your ability to burn fat. (See the next chapter for more information on duration.)

Another factor is intensity, or level of effort exerted. Research has found that the higher the exercise intensity, the longer the metabolism stays elevated afterwards.[3] (The next chapter discusses exercise intensity in depth.)

The type of exercise you do affects caloric afterburn too. Some studies have shown that strength training produces a greater caloric afterburn than even aerobic exercise. In a study of nine exercisers, researchers compared the metabolism-boosting power of strength training to cycling during a 40-minute workout session. What they found was interesting: Strength training produced a 36 percent higher increase in metabolism over cycling.[4]

# The Fat-Burning Power of Aerobic Exercise

Specific types of exercise have their own unique fat-burning benefits. Take aerobic exercise, for example. It burns fat in two special ways—by increasing fat-burning enzymes in the body and by improving oxygen delivery. Let's take a closer look at how these work.

Aerobic exercise increases your production of special enzymes that break down fat and enable the body to use fat as an energy source. You need higher levels of those enzymes if you want to get lean.

Aerobic exercise also improves your ability to process oxygen and deliver it to body cells. But how does this relate to fat-burning? Fatty acids

drawn from stored fat are the largest reservoir of fuel we have. In fact, normal-weight people have about 100,000 calories worth of stored fat on their bodies—roughly enough to power 200 hours of hard running. However, fat is not converted as easily to energy as carbohydrate is. The reason has to do with oxygen. The chemical reactions involved in converting carbohydrates to energy don't require oxygen. Therefore, energy can be supplied very rapidly if needed. But for fat to be burned as energy, oxygen is required, and the conversion process is a little more complicated.[5]

Well-trained aerobically fit people, however, burn fat very easily. Their bodies are efficient at delivering oxygen to muscle cells. The more oxygen these cells can get, the better the body can burn fatty acids for energy.

You can improve your own oxygen delivery system with a regular aerobic exercise program. Aerobic exercise enhances oxygen delivery in two major ways: (1) by increasing the network of blood vessels that feed muscle tissue with oxygen and nutrients; and (2) by conditioning the heart to deliver more blood with each beat. So the better conditioned you are aerobically, the more fat you can burn.

# The Fat-Burning Power of Strength Training

Strength training helps add muscle. The more muscle you have, the faster your metabolism. A faster metabolism translates into greater fat-burning potential.

The Swimsuit Lean program motivated Dana P. to incorporate strength training into her lifestyle full-time. As a result, she was able to gain a full pound of muscle during the 30-day period.

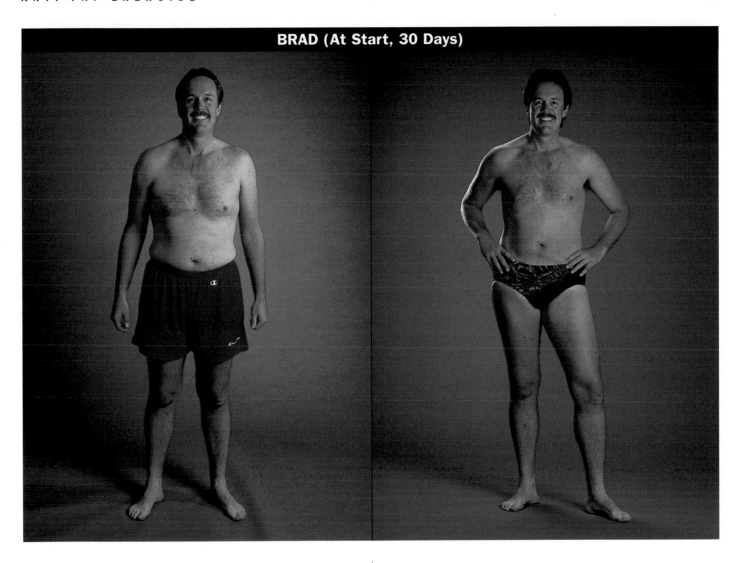

**BRAD (At Start, 30 Days)**

What will that mean for her long-term? A major effect on fat-burning, to be sure. As I noted in an earlier chapter, adding just one pound of muscle to your body helps you burn an additional 18,000 to 25,000 calories a year.

Most people who take up strength training for the first time love the results. Says Cindy S.: "Before starting the program, I was a very sporadic exerciser. I would work out several days per week for a couple of months and then stop exercising for a couple of months. At the times I did exercise, it consisted mainly of aerobic exercise with just a tiny bit of strength training. As a result of the Swimsuit Lean program, I began incorporating strength training into my routine. It has the potential to change the shape of the body tremendously. I noticed results in my shape just from weight training two times a week on the program."

Adds Dyan K.: "Strength training gives me the confidence to break out of the stereotypical idea that women have to be weak, frail, and inhibited. Strength training makes me feel more physically fit, as well as emotionally fit. I feel more independent and capable."

So start strength training! If you don't, you could jeopardize your metabolism. Unless you strength train, you could lose about a half a pound of muscle a year.[7]

# Do Both to Burn More

Want to dramatically burn fat by exercising? Do both types of exercise—aerobics *and* strength training. You'll multiply your fat-burning results, trim off inches, reshape your body, and dramatically improve your strength and endurance.

With strength training, you can firm up muscle underneath flabby areas. The routines in Chapter 18 include instructions on how to spot-shape troublesome areas—those bare-body areas like abs and thighs that hang out of your bathing suit. Granted, those locations where you have the most fat are genetically determined and hormonally controlled. Men, for example, tend to deposit fat around the waist, whereas women store it in the hips and thighs. Thigh fat is the toughest to burn because certain fat-mobilizing hormones there are less active. Consequently, the fat is more difficult to metabolize.

Even so, you can lower your overall percentage of body fat by exercising aerobically. The combination of aerobics and strength training helps you completely restructure your body.

After starting the Swimsuit Lean workout, don't be surprised if it looks as if your weight loss on the scale is happening at a snail's pace. As you develop lean muscle tissue and lose body fat, you'll lose inches along with pounds. And you may even gain weight—but it will be lean muscular weight. In the mirror, though, you'll appear trimmer, firmer, and more defined—exactly the way you want to look in your swimsuit.

# Did You Know That ...

There are other benefits attached to the recommended Swimsuit Lean workout, besides fat-burning. For example:

### HEART HEALTH

Regular exercise (both aerobic exercise and strength training) cuts your risk for cardiovascular disease by lowering cholesterol, reducing body fat, improving circulation, and lowering blood pressure. Exercise decreases your resting heart rate, which means your heart doesn't have to work so hard to pump blood when you're at rest. It also

## TABLE 13-1
### General Benefits of Exercise

| | |
|---|---|
| **Heart health** | Significantly reduces the risk of heart disease |
| **Stroke prevention** | Significantly reduces the risk of stroke. |
| **Diabetes (Type II)** | Protects against developing the disease and reduces insulin needs in those who have it |
| **High blood pressure** | Greatly normalized by exercise |
| **Muscles** | Increases metabolically active lean tissue |
| **Bones** | Reduces the risk of developing osteoporosis by stimulating the production of bone cells |
| **Joints** | Preserves function, mobility, and flexibility; protects joints, muscles, and bones against injury; guards against low-back pain |
| **Obesity** | Encourages the loss of body fat and the long-term maintenance of that loss |
| **Mental health** | Helps fight stress, anxiety, and depression; improves body image and well-being |
| **Family health** | Sets a positive example for children and encourages them to be active |

turns up the stroke volume of your heart (the amount of blood pumped out each heart beat). In short, exercise helps your heart do its job more efficiently.

## HEALTHY BLOOD

Dangerous levels of blood fats and cholesterol can zoom with poor health habits, increasing the risk of heart disease. Exercise counters these problems by increasing levels of good cholesterol in the body and stimulating circulation.

## BLOOD PRESSURE CONTROL

When your weight goes up, so does your blood pressure. Conversely, drop a few pounds, and your blood pressure drops too. The 30 Days to Swimsuit Lean Program is a fun approach to blood pressure control.

## BONE HEALTH

After astronauts go into space for any length of time, they lose bone mass because of the weight-less-ness of the environment. The same thing can happen to you from a lack of force put on your muscles—in other words, inactivity.

One of the best ways to prevent bone loss is to strength train regularly. Strength training builds muscle mass *and* bone mass—by stimulating the bone to produce new cells. Other forms of exercise such as walking, step aerobics, calisthenics, bicycling—any movement that gets your muscles working against gravity— offer protection against bone loss, too.

If you lose too much bone over your lifetime, you could develop osteoporosis, a crippling bone-thinning disease that affects mostly women. It's the reason behind many telltale signs of aging that appear in your fifties and sixties—loss of height, aches and pains, a curved back, immobility, and limbs that break easily.

There are many risk factors for osteoporosis besides inactivity—being female, early menopause, chronically low intake of calcium, family history, smoking, and excessive use of alcohol. Most of these risk factors can be controlled. Put another way, you can prevent or at least retard the development of osteoporosis, no matter what your age. And regular exercise, along with a healthy diet, is one way to do it.

## NERVOUS SYSTEM

Exercise is a natural tranquilizer, reducing stress, anxiety, and depression. What's more, exercise helps you sleep more soundly.

These and other benefits of exercise are summarized in Table 13-1.

In the next several chapters, you'll find exact instructions on what exercise to select, how to work out, spot-shape your body, and accelerate your fat loss through the proper combination of aerobics and strength training.

# Chapter 14
## Choosing the Right Exercise

A recent report issued by the U.S. Surgeon General said that more than 60 percent of American adults are not getting enough exercise every day to stay healthy, and 25 percent do not exercise at all. Citing numerous scientific studies, this first-ever report noted that Americans are becoming a nation of couch potatoes, at risk for an increasing number of life-shortening illnesses such as heart disease, high blood pressure, colon cancer, and diabetes. Also according to the report, an estimated 250,000 deaths in the U.S. each year can be linked to a lack of exercise.[1]

Why aren't more people exercising? One reason may be that a lot of us think exercise is a chore, another requirement on the long list of ways "to get healthy." But let's flashback for a moment: Remember when you were a kid? Weren't you active most of the time, climbing trees, playing ball, swimming, chasing your friends in a game of tag? And wasn't it fun?

To make exercise a part of your life, you have to enjoy it. It has to be fun, an activity that brings back the kid in you, or at least the spirit of enjoyment. One way to do that is to make sure you choose the right type of exercise, particularly aerobic exercise.

The first step is to educate yourself about the special advantages of each type of aerobic exercise. To help you, here is an at-a-glance chart (Table 14-1) explaining various aerobic exercise options, their benefits, and the level of effort you need to put forth to reap those benefits.

## TABLE 14-1

# *Aerobic Exercise Options*

| EXERCISE | SPECIAL ADVANTAGES | PERFORMANCE TIPS | HOW MUCH, HOW HARD |
|---|---|---|---|
| Walking | • Good for beginners<br>• Low rate of injury<br>• A do-anywhere activity<br>• Helps shed abdominal fat | • Walk heel to toe.<br>• Walk at a brisk pace.<br>• Maintain good posture.<br>• Pump your arms in a swinging motion. | • Try to increase your distance or duration each time you walk.<br>• Increase your pace so that you're covering the same distance in less time.<br>• 30 to 45 minutes each session* |
| Running/ Jogging | • Excellent for fat-burning<br>• Helps shed abdominal fat<br>• Strengthens & tones leg muscles | • Take heel to toe strides.<br>• Run on smooth surfaces (grassy or cushioned tracks).<br>• Maintain an erect position with head up.<br>• Breathe normally.<br>• Wear proper shoes. | • Pick up your pace, increase your duration, or increase your frequency.<br>• 30 to 45 minutes each session* |
| Swimming | • Enjoyable for those who like the water<br>• Well-suited for people with joint problems<br>• Works all body muscles | • Master the key strokes. | • Perform as much non-stop swimming as you can.<br>• Add laps gradually each week.<br>• 30 to 45 minutes each session* |
| Biking | • Helps build thigh muscles | • Make sure bicycle is fitted to your frame.<br>• Wear proper headgear. | • Pick up your pace, increase your duration, or increase your frequency.<br>• 30 to 45 minutes each session* |
| Aerobic Dance | • Enjoyable for those who like music and dance<br>• Works the whole body<br>• Various skill levels available | • The workout should include a warm-up, an aerobic segment that's 20 to 30 minutes long, and a cool-down consisting of walking or light jogging. | • Start with a beginner's class, then progress to a more advanced level.<br>• 45 to 60 minutes each class |

*See Chapter 13 for the recommended number of daily aerobic sessions.

## TABLE 14-1 continued
# *Aerobic Exercise Options*

| EXERCISE | SPECIAL ADVANTAGES | PERFORMANCE TIPS | HOW MUCH, HOW HARD |
|---|---|---|---|
| Treadmill | • Strengthens and tones the thighs, buttocks, and calves<br>• Rated as the most effective aerobic exercise when exercisers run on it | • Follow manufacturer's safety instructions.<br>• Walk, jog, or run at a pace that keeps up with the belt. | • Try to increase your distance or duration each time you use the machine.<br>• Use intensity-building features of the machine.<br>• 30 to 45 minutes each session* |
| Stationary Cycle | • Appropriate for overweight exercisers<br>• Easy on the back<br>• Strengthens and tones the thighs | • Follow manufacturer's safety instructions. | • Try to increase your distance or duration each time you use the machine.<br>• Use intensity-building features of the machine.<br>• 30 to 45 minutes each session* |
| Stairclimber | • Strengthens and tones the thighs, buttocks, and calves | • Follow manufacturer's safety instructions.<br>• Resist the temptation to rest on the handrails. | • Try to increase your distance or duration each time you use the machine.<br>• Use intensity-building features of the machine.<br>• 30 to 45 minutes each session* |
| Rowing Machine | • Strengthens and tones the upper body | • Follow manufacturer's safety instructions.<br>• Keep back straight while rowing. | • Try to increase your distance or duration each time you use the machine.<br>• Use intensity-building features of the machine.<br>• 30 to 45 minutes each session* |

*See Chapter 13 for the recommended number of daily aerobic sessions.

The exercise you choose should match your personality and your lifestyle. To help you in your selection, let's have a little fun by taking the following quizzes. If you've exercised for some time now, these quizzes will affirm your exercise choices, or perhaps show you some new possibilities. For newcomers to exercise, you'll find out right away which activities are best for you.

# Your Workout Personality

What kind of "workout personality" do you have? My co-author Maggie Greenwood-Robinson devised this quiz while researching exercise motivation and the personality factors related to it.

Here's a list of 40 adjectives. Circle the numbers of the **twelve** you can honestly apply to yourself.

| | |
|---|---|
| 1. orderly | 21. reserved |
| 2. spontaneous | 22. talkative |
| 3. introverted | 23. logical |
| 4. open | 24. fickle |
| 5. methodical | 25. usually serious |
| 6. easily bored | 26. exuberant |
| 7. tidy | 27. organized |
| 8. amiable | 28. capricious |
| 9. quiet | 29. private |
| 10. flexible | 30. easygoing |
| 11. disciplined | 31. resolute |
| 12. lazy | 32. casual |
| 13. modest | 33. systematic |
| 14. outgoing | 34. friendly |
| 15. rigid | 35. unimaginative |
| 16. impulsive | 36. emotional |
| 17. self-conscious | 37. prompt |
| 18. warm | 38. adaptable |
| 19. analytical | 39. evasive |
| 20. versatile | 40. helpful |

**Scoring:** If you circled mostly odd-numbered adjectives, your personality is best suited to solitary exercise, such as strength training, walking, exercising at home. You may not enjoy competitive exercises or ones in which a high degree of skill is required. If you pursue competitive activities, you are inclined toward individual sports such as racquetball or tennis, rather than team activities. You prefer working out alone as opposed to working out with a group or in a class. Your chance of exercise success is highest when you have a fairly well-regimented routine to follow—with specific exercises and measurable goals.

If you circled mostly even-numbered adjectives, you like to work out with others, often in classes and at exercise facilities. When performing a solitary activity such as strength training, you need to change your exercises frequently because you become bored easily. In fact, you need to vary your total exercise routine a lot—by walking one day, biking the next, and so forth. Aerobic "cross-training" is a good idea too. Start out with 10 to 15 minutes on a treadmill, followed by 10 to 15 minutes on a stairclimbing machine, and end with 10 to 15 minutes on a rowing machine.

# Exercise Selection

If you're going to do it (exercise), then you've got to stick to it! Many lifestyle factors can influence your stick-to-it-ive-ness, from affordability to convenience. Quiz #2 will help you identify those activities best suited to your lifestyle.

**Scoring:** Under each category (i.e. It will be fun for me, I can afford it, etc.) rate the exercise according to the following numerical system:

**1** = Not at all
**3** = Somewhat
**5** = For the most part

Tally up your score for each activity, and you'll have a good idea of which exercise will work best for you.

| EXERCISE QUIZ #2 | | | | |
|---|---|---|---|---|
| Exercise | It will be fun for me. | I can do it successfully. | It is convenient. | I can afford it. | Totals |
| Walking | | | | | |
| Running/ Jogging | | | | | |
| Swimming | | | | | |
| Biking | | | | | |
| Aerobic Dance | | | | | |
| Treadmill | | | | | |
| Stationary Cycle | | | | | |
| Stairclimber | | | | | |
| Rowing Machine | | | | | |
| Strength Training (Gym) | | | | | |
| Strength Training (Home) | | | | | |

# Staying Motivated

By now, you know that exercise is a key to becoming swimsuit lean. But do you ever find yourself making excuses about not getting to the gym or hopping on the exercise bike? One of the biggest excuses is time. "I can't find the time today." "Something came up." "It's too late." If you find yourself falling into time traps, let me suggest:

- Schedule your workouts in your weekly calendar or daytimer, just as you would other important appointments.
- Keep your gym gear in your car, so you'll be ready to work out, anywhere and anytime.
- Simplify your life and save time by doing your aerobics at home. Walk, jog, run—or invest in home workout equipment, particularly aerobic machines like a stationary bicycle, treadmill, or stairclimber. By working out at home, you don't have to spend time commuting to and from a gym. Home workouts adapt to your schedule.
- Get your aerobics in early, as the Swimsuit Lean program recommends. Not only have we observed that you burn more fat, you also get your workout out of the way early in the day.

Finding out what works for other people is motivating as well. To help you, here are some comments on exercise motivation from several of our Swimsuit Lean participants:

"Motivation is easier the longer you stay with it. Just thinking of the alternative is all the motivation I need."

—**Dyan K.**

"You have to finally get to the point where you're ready to make some real changes in your life. I have to try to give it to God and ask Him for the strength. Don't ever think you're beyond being changed."

—**Tracy S.**

"My motivation comes from results! It is fun to notice the changes…going another block, running a little farther, lifting a little more weight, or getting more reps. I never would have believed I'd look forward to getting up at 5 a.m. to walk. But when I don't, I really miss it. Exercising helps me start the day with so much more energy."

—**Larry K.**

"One great motivator I've found in exercising is the energy you get. Once you get out of the habit, you go back to feeling tired, sluggish, and unmotivated."

—**Cindy S.**

"In military service, I used to be motivated by military requirements to maintain a certain level of fitness, but even that didn't stop my slow, downward spiral. I finally got disgusted with how I looked and felt and knew I had to start exercising again to turn things around. What motivates me now is my muscular development and the positive responses I get from others. It's also important to find a variety of exercise activities you enjoy, and then do them at a convenient time."

—**Jerry M.**

"The one thing that keeps me on my running schedule is having a training partner. It's like an appointment—you have to be there! As for weight training, the quick results alone keep me going back for more. With exercise and the eating plan, I've lost 5.65 percent body fat."

—**Beverly J.**

**BEVERLY J. (At Start, 30 Days, 60 Days)**

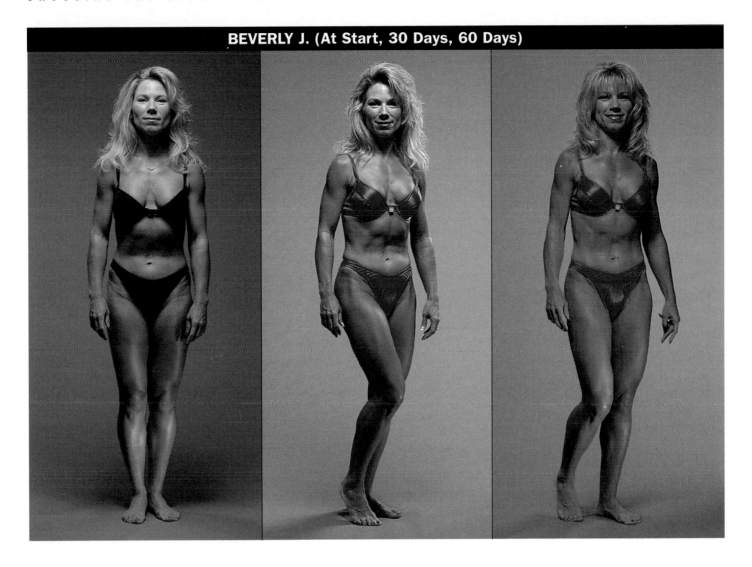

# Keep an Exercise Log

One practice that helps people stick to the Swimsuit Lean program is keeping an exercise log. Simply write down the exercises you do, including your aerobics, in a simple notebook, noting the day and time. Then track the number of repetitions you perform (for strength training) and the duration of your aerobic activity. Each time you exercise, try to do more until you've reached a comfortable level. Your log thus becomes a reflection of your exercise progress.

To help you, on the following page is a sample exercise log you can use to chart your progress.

**SWIMSUIT LEAN WORKOUT LOG**          Date:

**Resting Heart Rate:**                **Target Heart Rate:**

| EXERCISE | SETS/REPS | POUNDAGE |
|----------|-----------|----------|
|          |           |          |
|          |           |          |
|          |           |          |
|          |           |          |
|          |           |          |
|          |           |          |
|          |           |          |
|          |           |          |
|          |           |          |
|          |           |          |
|          |           |          |
|          |           |          |
|          |           |          |
|          |           |          |
|          |           |          |

| AEROBICS | TIME/DISTANCE | TIME OF DAY |
|----------|---------------|-------------|
|          |               |             |
|          |               |             |
|          |               |             |
|          |               |             |
|          |               |             |
|          |               |             |
|          |               |             |
|          |               |             |
|          |               |             |
|          |               |             |
|          |               |             |

# Chapter 15
## *Fat Loss Accelerators*

*I*f there were bonafide ways to speed up your fat loss and encourage your body to tap into its fat stores more rapidly, wouldn't you want to try them? Of course! What follows is an explanation of certain techniques that can help you accelerate your fat loss.

## Increase the "Intensity" of Your Exercise

Intensity refers to the level of effort you exert during exercise. Higher-intensity exercise helps you get leaner and more toned much faster.

How do you know if you're exercising intensely enough? There are a couple of ways to tell. With aerobic exercise, you should be breathing hard but still be able to carry on a conversation. This indicates that your body is processing a significant amount of oxygen. When more oxygen is "extracted" by your muscles, more stored fat and carbohydrate can be used to supply energy.

Another way to determine aerobic intensity is by monitoring your heart rate. For best results, you should exercise at a level sufficient enough to raise your heart rate to 70 to 85 percent or higher of your maximum heart rate (MHR). MHR is expressed as 220 minus your age. For example, suppose you're 40 years old, and you start an aerobic exercise program. Your maximum heart rate is 180 (220 - 40). You should work out at such an intensity that your heart reaches between 126 and 153 beats a minute (70 to 85 percent of 180 beats per minute = .70 x 180 = 126, or .80 x 180 = 153).

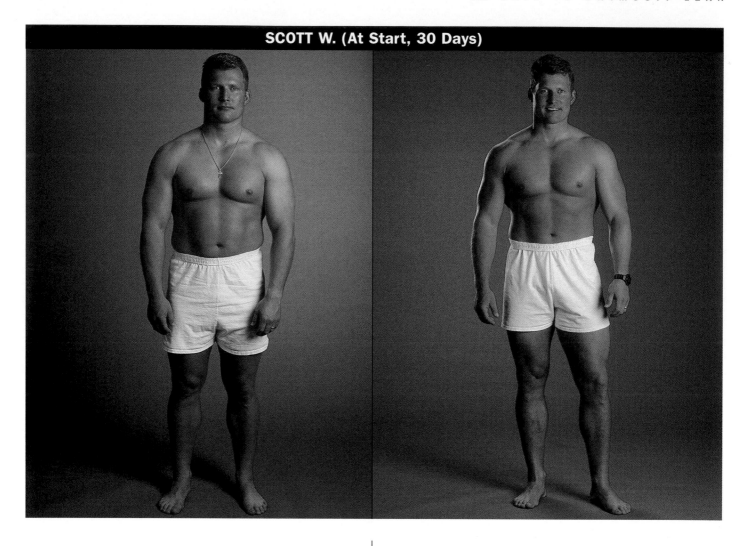

**SCOTT W. (At Start, 30 Days)**

If you're a newcomer to aerobic exercise, start out in the lower end of your range. Gradually increase your intensity so that you reach the higher end of your range as your body becomes more aerobically fit.

Higher-intensity aerobic exercise burns more fat. To illustrate what I mean, let's look at two examples. First, suppose you walk for about 45 minutes at about three miles per hour, elevating your heart rate to about 65 percent of its maximum—a moderate level of intensity. At this intensity, you're burning a total of 216 calories—108 calories from carbohydrates and 108 calories from fat.

In the second example, you pick up your pace by walking four miles per hour and elevating your heart rate to 75 percent of its maximum. In the same 45-minute period, you'll burn a total of 288 calories—176 calories from carbohydrates and 112 calories from fat. So at the higher intensity level, more of your energy comes from fat (112 fat calories versus 108 calories).[1]

# How to Increase Your Intensity

### ■ *Aerobic Exercise Machines*

Aerobic exercise machines are immensely popular—and for good reason. Their high-tech bells and whistles make exercising fun and challenging. You can watch your intensity build in dot patterns on the screen in front of you, punch a button to see how many calories you've burned, or check the speed at which you're moving. It's hard to get bored.

To burn more fat, strive to increase your intensity on these machines. You can do this easily by choosing the appropriate program and level of effort. Most machines offer three basic programs—manual, random, or hills. Manual programs maintain a consistent workout, without any variation in intensity or speed, unless you manually change these options. Random programs keep you guessing; one moment you're speeding up, the next you're slowing down. With hills, you can choose any number of hill profiles—from steep to steady climbs.

As for intensity level, most aerobic exercise machines let you choose from level 1 to level 20. The higher numbers signify the more intense routines. Beginners to these machines should work out at a level between 1 and 4 for at least 20 minutes each time. Try to add five extra minutes each workout (or at your own pace—gauge how you feel). After about two weeks of increasing your duration, increase the level by one point and continue to do so each week.

If you're already more conditioned aerobically, you may be able to start at the mid-range levels of intensity (levels 5 - 8). Begin with 30 minute workouts the first week, then increase your duration by five minutes each workout (or at your own pace—gauge how you feel). By the second week, adjust your level of intensity upward as your duration increases. Work up to a comfortable intensity level. Some people like to mix and match their workouts, using several different machines in a cross-training approach to aerobics. For example:

- 10 minutes on the treadmill
- 10 minutes on a rowing machine
- 10 minutes on a stationary bicycle
- 10 minutes on a stairclimbing machine

If you do this, keep in mind that intensity varies from machine to machine. What feels difficult at level 8 on a stairclimber might feel quite easy on a stationary bicycle.

## ■ Strength Training

Intensity in strength training refers primarily to the demand you place on your muscles—in other words, how much weight you lift or how many repetitions of an exercise you do. For greater intensity, you must challenge your muscles to lift more weight or do more repetitions each time you work out. Working your muscles hard ultimately leads to more lean tissue and less body fat.

# Shift Your Body into a Fat-Burning Mode

### Perform Aerobics after Strength Training

You can shift your body into a fat-burning mode faster if you perform your aerobic exercise *after* strength training. Lifting weights causes your body to draw on muscle glycogen for fuel. During a 30 to 45-minute training session, you can use up a lot of glycogen. Afterwards, your body is glycogen-needy—the perfect time to start your aerobics. Theoretically, your body then starts drawing on fatty acids for energy during the aerobics. You'll burn more fat and get leaner as a result.

# Lose More Fat

### ■ Increase The Duration of Your Aerobic Workout

For various reasons, some people just can't push for higher intensities. If you're one of them, don't despair! Simply increase the duration of your aerobic workout. The longer you work out aerobically—45 minutes or longer—the more fat you'll burn.

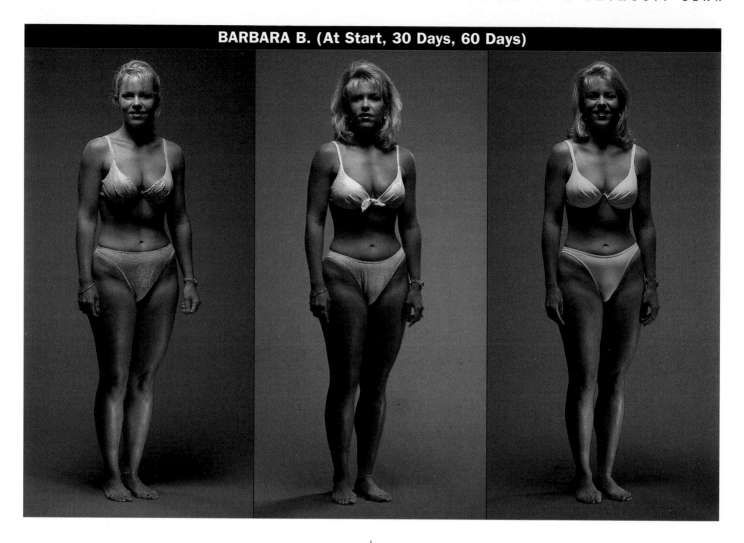

**BARBARA B. (At Start, 30 Days, 60 Days)**

■ *Increase The Frequency of Your Workouts*

You can burn more fat by increasing the number of times you work out each week. If you've been exercising aerobically three times a week, gradually work up to four or five times a week. You'll burn more calories. Many of those calories will be fat calories, especially if you're working out at higher intensities.

Scott W. increased both the duration and frequency of his aerobic activity—up to four times a week for 30 to 45 minutes each time. Scott's before-and-after photos on page 100 show the visible results of his efforts.

# Take Gradual Steps

It can be tempting to work out harder and longer or add more exercise sessions—and do it right away. But proceed with caution, or you could hurt yourself. Make small upward increments in intensity, duration, and frequency, and you'll be gratified by what you can accomplish. Barbara B., who lost nearly 3 percent body fat on Swimsuit Lean, is a good example. Several years ago, she complained to her husband about her overweight condition. He told her to do something about it. So she started a running program. At first, Barbara could run only half a mile. But she kept at it, and three years later, she was running six or more miles every time she hit the track.

# Chapter 16
## Rules for Safe Exercise

To make your exercise experience safe and effective, be sure to follow these general guidelines:

## Aerobic Exercise

1. Have a physical examination, including a stress test, before beginning a program of aerobic exercise.

2. If you have not done aerobic exercise prior to Swimsuit Lean, start gradually with 20 minutes at first and add five minutes each time afterwards, as your endurance improves.

3. Wear comfortable yet sturdy footwear suited for the particular type of aerobics you choose. Also, wear comfortable, loose-fitting clothes that suit the temperature outside or indoors, depending on where you exercise.

4. To improve your level of cardiovascular fitness and fat-burning potential, try to keep your heart rate elevated to 70 to 85 percent of its maximum for at least 15 to 20 minutes.

5. Begin each aerobic workout with a warm-up and finish off with a cool-down. These can consist of five minutes of walking, light jogging, or other low-intensity work. Aerobic exercise machines have warm-up and cool-down periods already built into the exercise program.

**6** Breathe naturally and comfortably while exercising. Holding your breath will rob you of energy and could cause fainting.

**7** Be sure you are well-hydrated prior to exercising. Drink at least two glasses of water a few hours before aerobic exercise and a half glass about a half hour before your exercise session. It is also advisable to sip some water every 15 or 20 minutes while exercising, particularly if you perspire heavily.

**8** If you feel faint, dizzy, or experience any untoward reaction, stop exercising immediately and seek medical attention.

# Strength Training

**1** If you're past the age of 30, have been inactive for some period of time, or have a health problem, you should undergo a physical examination prior to beginning the Swimsuit Lean workout.

**2** Work out with weights at least twice a week, on non-consecutive days.

**3** Try to exercise each muscle group to "fatigue"—the point at which you feel you can no longer complete another repetition. This effectively challenges your muscles and stimulates their growth. Exercising to fatigue is an advanced technique; not everyone will be able to work at this intensity.

**4** To stimulate fat-burning, rest approximately 30 to 45 seconds between each exercise. This abbreviated rest interval provides enough of an aerobic effect to assist in fat-burning. For muscular development, it's better to rest one to two minutes.

**5** Start with a poundage that lets you learn the exercise correctly and comfortably before progressing to heavier weights.

**6** Breathe comfortably and naturally as you lift weights. Never hold your breath during an exercise. Doing so will build up dangerous pressure, impeding blood flow to and from your brain, and could cause a fainting spell.

**7** Proper exercise form is essential. Try to concentrate on the body part you are working, without jerking, bending your back unnecessarily, or swaying your body. Such motion deprives the muscles of proper stimulation.

**8** Move the weight through a full range of motion.

**9** When you lift a weight, do it slowly—about three or four seconds. Lower it even more slowly. Never lift weights quickly. Doing so will only harm your joints and keep your muscles from being properly stimulated.

**⑩** Wear clothing that allows your limbs a full range of motion and is appropriate for the temperature in the gym.

**⑪** Never attempt to train alone on exercises such as the bench press that require a spotter. Normally this is not a problem if you work out at a gym where there are groups of people exercising. But if working out at home, have someone present while you exercise.

**⑫** Use safety equipment while strength training, including collars on dumbbells and barbells and catch racks on pressing benches and squat racks.

**⑬** Perform a warm-up set for each muscle group you are working. A warm-up set consists of 12 to 15 repetitions with a light poundage, or a poundage that is roughly one-half what you would use on your working set. (A repetition or rep is the number of times an exercise is performed. A set is a series of repetitions.)

**⑭** Beginners should perform two sets of 12 to 15 repetitions. Experienced strength trainers can perform three or more sets of 12 to 15 repetitions.

**⑮** Practice good gym housekeeping. Return plates and weights to their proper places as soon as you are finished using them. This will prevent tripping hazards in the gym.

**⑯** Stay informed about strength training. The more educated you are about strength training and other forms of exercise, the better progress you'll make and the fewer injuries you'll experience.

**⑰** If you feel faint, dizzy, or experience any untoward reaction, stop exercising immediately and seek medical attention.

# General Pointers

By exercising regularly, you're doing your body and your health a huge favor. Exercise is a privilege, not a chore. With that in mind, here are a few general tips to keep you on track:

**❶** Set goals for your exercise program—in terms of intensity, duration, frequency, and sets and repetitions (for strength training). But make sure the goals you set for yourself are realistic.

**❷** Acknowledge each gain you make, even if it doesn't seem significant.

**❸** Avoid comparing yourself to anyone else. Your biochemistry, body type, and metabolism are as individual as you are.

# Rest and Recovery

Sleep is essential to the body's ability to restore its muscles and energy systems. The heart, especially, needs sufficient rest. It pumps enough blood each day to fill a railroad car.

Muscles need a minimum of 48 hours of rest before being exercised again. It's during this time that actual muscle strengthening and toning take place. To allow for adequate recovery, never work the same muscle groups two days in a row.

Proper nutrition also allows your body to repair itself following workouts so that lean muscle can be developed.

# Chapter 17
## Swimsuit Lean Exercises

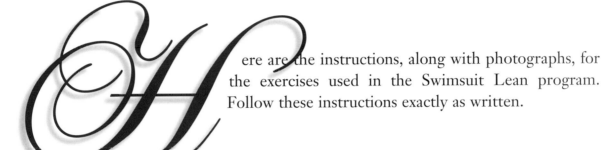

ere are the instructions, along with photographs, for the exercises used in the Swimsuit Lean program. Follow these instructions exactly as written.

- ■ Thigh Exercises

- ■ Buttocks/Hamstring Exercises

- ■ Chest Exercises

- ■ Back Exercises

- ■ Shoulder Exercises

- ■ Triceps Exercises

- ■ Biceps Exercises

- ■ Abdominal Exercises

- ■ Lower Leg Exercises

**THIGH EXERCISE**

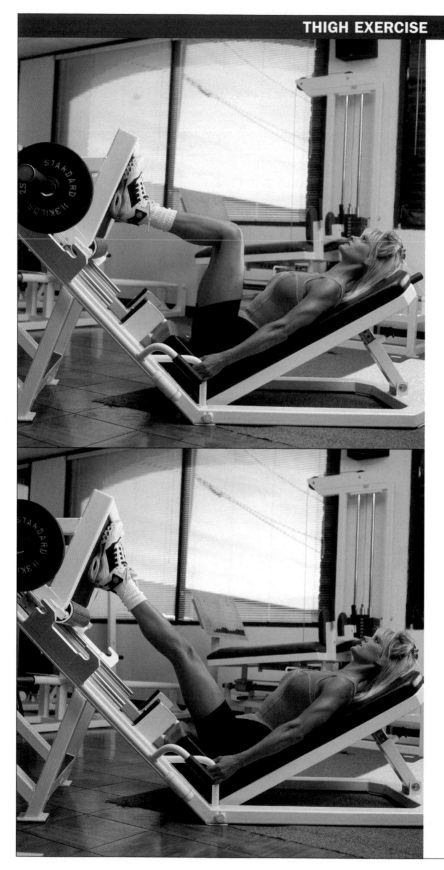

# Leg Press

Position yourself in the leg press machine so that your back lies against the bench of the machine.

Place your hands on the grips, which are usually at your side.

Place your feet on the footplate about hip-width apart. Push the footplate up slightly to release the safety catch. Do not lock your knee joints at any time during the exercise.

Bend your knees toward your chest. Descend only to the point of 90 degrees and not farther. Your knees should never touch your chest.

Concentrate on pushing with your heels, rather than the balls of your feet. Keep your knees in line with your feet.

Repeat the exercise for the recommended number of sets and repetitions.

**THIGH EXERCISE**

# Lunge

Place your legs in a scissor position as shown in the photograph.

Keeping proper postural alignment, lower body straight down. Keep the front lower leg perpendicular to the floor. Do not let your knee go forward (see photograph).

At the bottom of the movement, your back knee should be within a few inches of the floor.

*Note: You may use dumbbells or a barbell for added resistance.*

Repeat the movement on the same leg for the required number of sets and repetitions.

Repeat the exercise on the other leg.

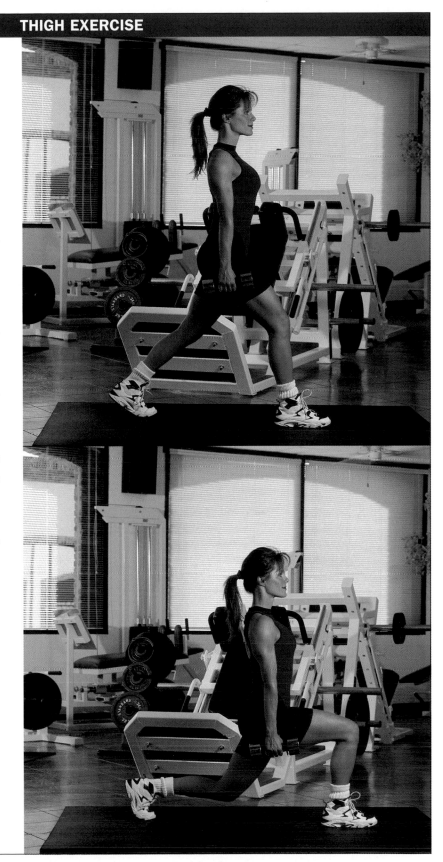

**THIGH EXERCISE**

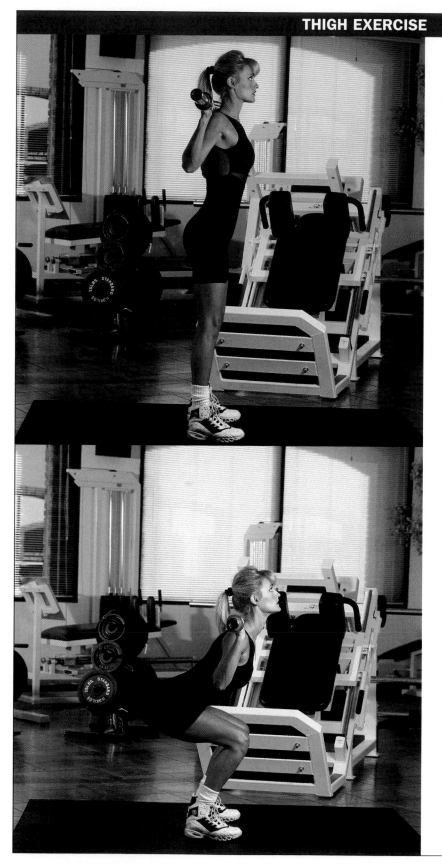

# Squat

This exercise should be performed with the use of a squat rack.

Before beginning the exercise, adjust the barbell on the rack to a comfortable position.

Position yourself under the bar so that the bar is resting on the back of your shoulders.

Maintaining proper postural alignment, slowly lower your body (while sitting back) to a point at which your thighs are parallel to the floor. (However, it is not necessary to go all the way to a parallel position to benefit from this exercise.

Slowly return to the starting position by straightening your legs.

Repeat the exercise for the recommended number of sets and repetitions.

**THIGH EXERCISE**

# Leg extension

Sit in the leg extension machine and hook your ankles under the padded roller.

Extend your legs upward in an arc. At the top, tense the muscles for a moment or two. Lower slowly to the starting position.

Repeat the exercise for the recommended number of sets and repetitions.

*Note: Some physical therapists are concerned that this movement may further aggravate pre-existing knee injuries.*

*Note: If you perform this exercise do not exceed a 60-degree range of motion.*

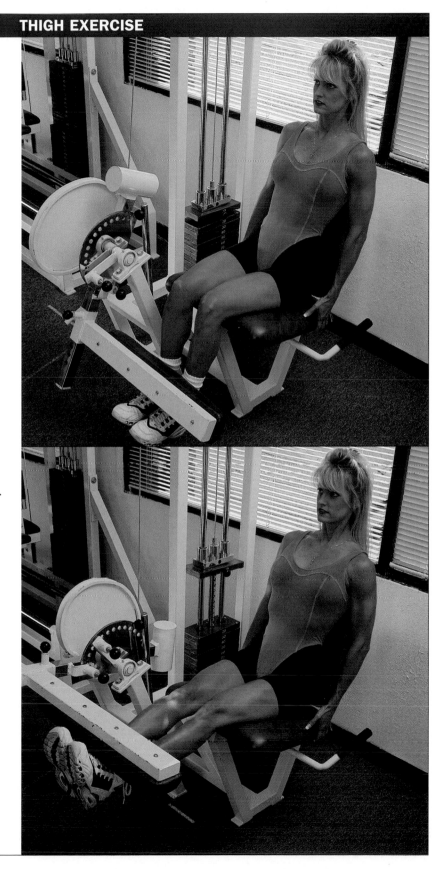

**THIGH EXERCISE**

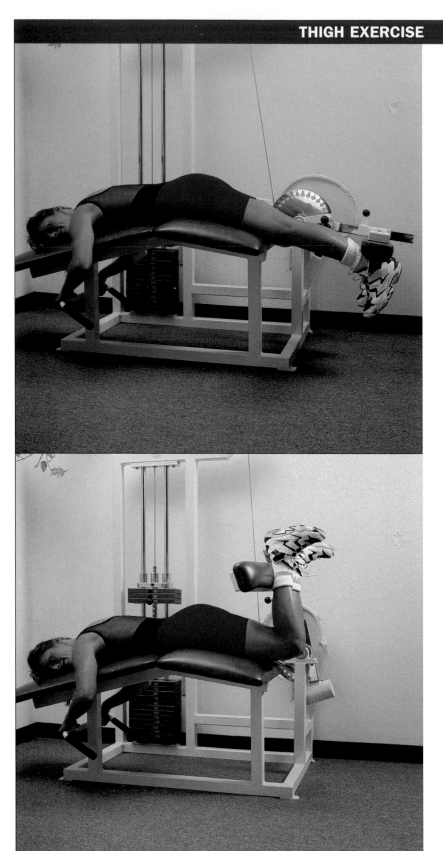

# Leg curl

Lie face down on the bench of the leg machine and take hold of the grips on either side. Your legs should be extended so that the edge of the bench is just above your knees. (Your kneecap should be positioned just beyond the edge of the bench, but not touching.)

Hook your ankles under the padded roller.

Flex your knees, bringing your lower legs toward your buttocks. Keep your hips pressed into the bench.

Slowly return to the starting position.

Repeat the exercise for the recommended number of sets and repetitions.

**THIGH EXERCISE**

# Hack squat

To perform this exercise, you will need a special machine called a hack slide, a popular piece of equipment found in most gyms and health clubs.

Step into the machine and face forward (with your back against the body of the machine).

Position yourself under the shoulder pad, and place your feet about hip-width apart, with your toes pointing slightly outward.

Release the safety latches, and slowly slide up and down by bending and straightening your knees. It is not necessary to descend lower than 90 degrees.

Perform the exercise for the recommended number of sets and repetitions.

An apparatus known as a "Smith machine" can also be used for this exercise.

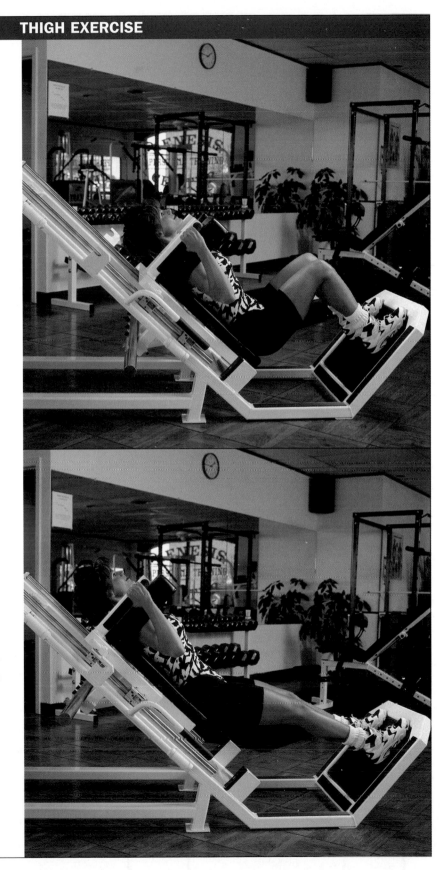

## BUTTOCKS/HAMSTRING EXERCISE

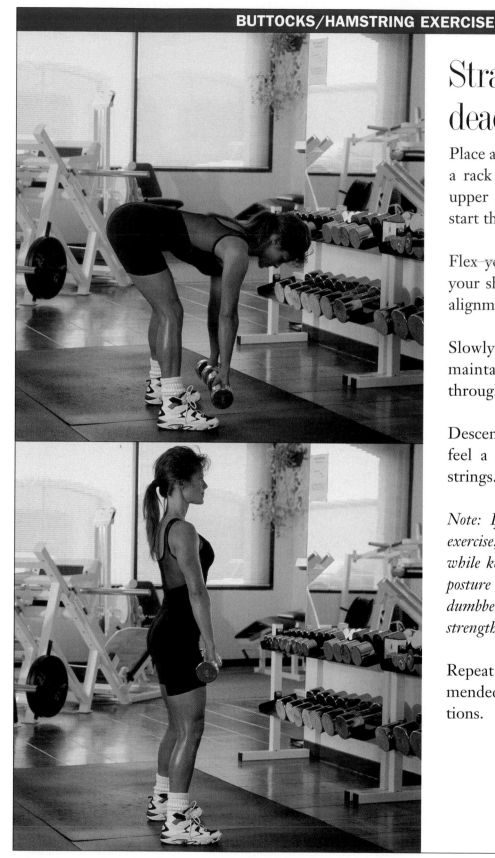

# Straight leg deadlift

Place a barbell or two dumbbells on a rack at a position between your upper thigh and hip level. Do not start this exercise from the floor.

Flex your knees slightly and keep your shoulders and back in proper alignment.

Slowly bend at the waist while maintaining proper posture throughout the exercise.

Descend to the point at which you feel a deep stretch in your hamstrings.

*Note: If you use dumbbells for this exercise, squat down to the weights while keeping your back in the proper posture and alignment; then grip the dumbbells and ascend upward using the strength of your legs, not your back.*

Repeat the exercise for the recommended number of sets and repetitions.

**CHEST EXERCISE**

# Bench press

Lie back on a flat exercise bench with your knees bent and your feet flat on the floor. Your back should maintain contact with the bench.

Have someone hand you the barbell, or lift it off the rack at the head of the bench. Take a shoulder-width grip on the bar, although grip width may vary from person to person. Hold the barbell over your shoulders with your arms extended. Slowly lower the barbell to your chest. Do not bounce at the bottom of the movement. Press the barbell upward to the starting position without locking your elbow joints. Tense your chest muscles.

Repeat the exercise for the recommended number of sets and repetitions.

*Strict form is critical. Beginners should practice the exercise with an empty bar to perfect proper technique. Try not to let the bar bounce off your chest after the lowering phase of the exercise. Bouncing could injure your chest and ribcage. Nor should you arch your back during the lift. This action could put dangerous pressure on your spine. To prevent arching, keep your feet flat on the floor and your back pressed close to the bench.*

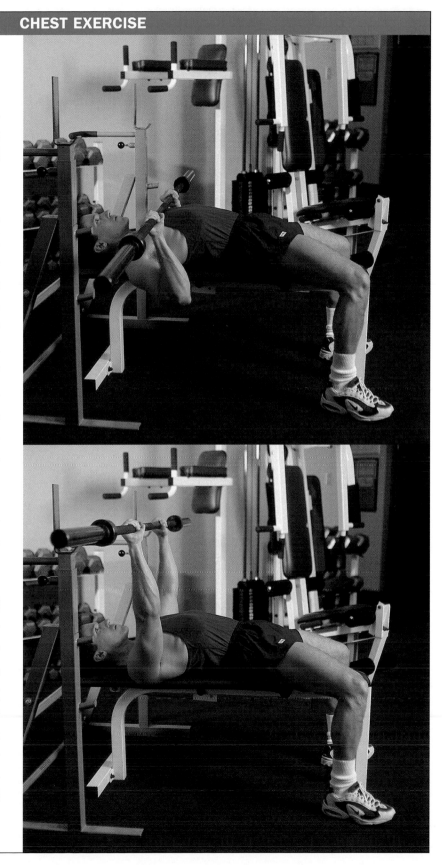

**CHEST EXERCISE**

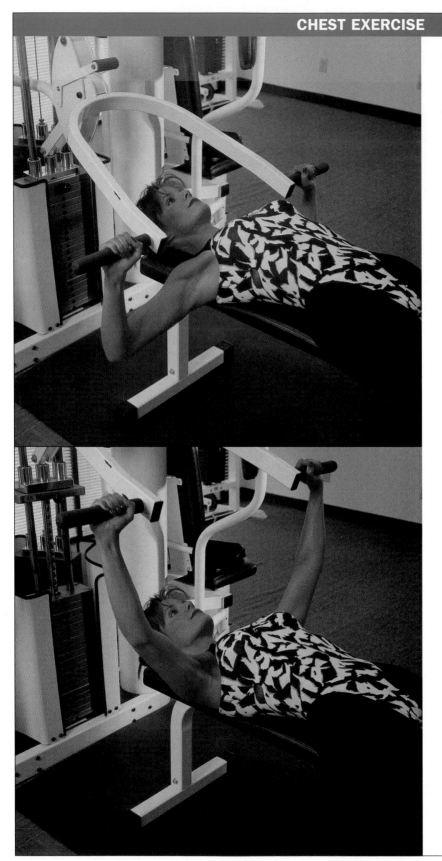

# Machine bench press

If you prefer machine training, bench press machines are an effective way to build and shape the chest. With some machines, you'll lie on your back; with others, you'll sit upright.

Either way, press the bar of the machine out but stop short of fully extending your arms. Then slowly bring the bar back, always emphasizing proper form.

Repeat the exercise for the recommended number of sets and repetitions.

**CHEST EXERCISE**

# Dumbbell fly

Lie back on a flat bench with your feet touching the floor.

Take a dumbbell in each hand and extend your arms to a position directly over your chest. The palms of your hands should be facing each other.

Slowly lower your arms out to your sides, getting a good stretch at the bottom of the exercise (as far as is comfortable). Then bring the weights back together (without letting them touch). Tense your chest muscles.

Return to the starting position, and repeat the exercise for the recommended number of sets and repetitions.

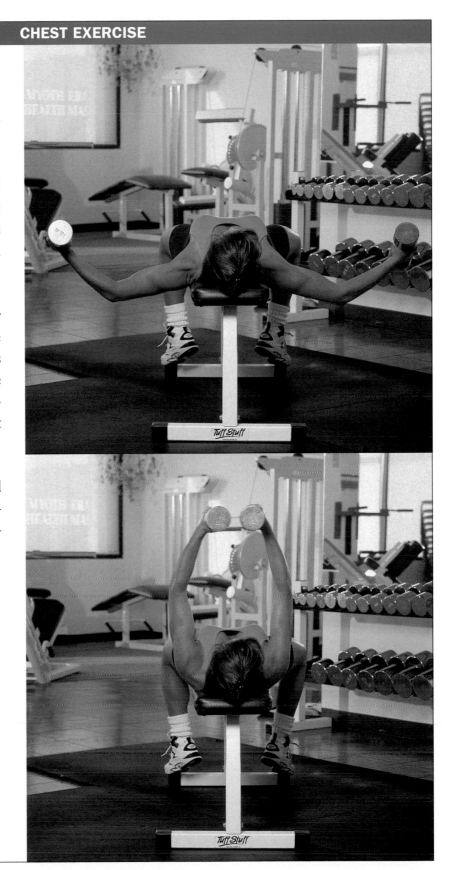

**BACK EXERCISE**

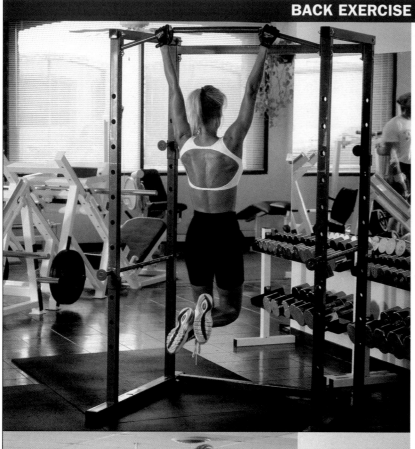

# Chins

To perform the chin-up, take an underhand grip (slightly less than shoulder-width) or an overhand grip (about shoulder-width) on the chinning bar.

Slowly hoist yourself up until your chin is just above the bar. Try to bring your chest to the bar.

Lower and repeat for as many repetitions as you can.

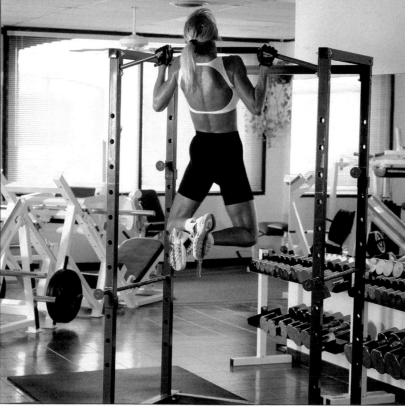

**BACK EXERCISE**

# Partner-assisted dumbbell pullover

Position your body crosswise to an exercise bench. Your upper back should rest on the bench, and your knees should be bent, as pictured.

Have your partner hand you a dumbbell so that you can execute a "cupping" grip, as pictured.

Bend your elbows slightly, and slowly bring the dumbbell back to a position behind your head. Keep your elbows slightly flexed. Strive for a good stretch at the bottom of the movement; however, stretch only as far as is comfortable. Do not bounce.

Return the dumbbell to the starting position, and repeat the exercise for the suggested number of sets and repetitions.

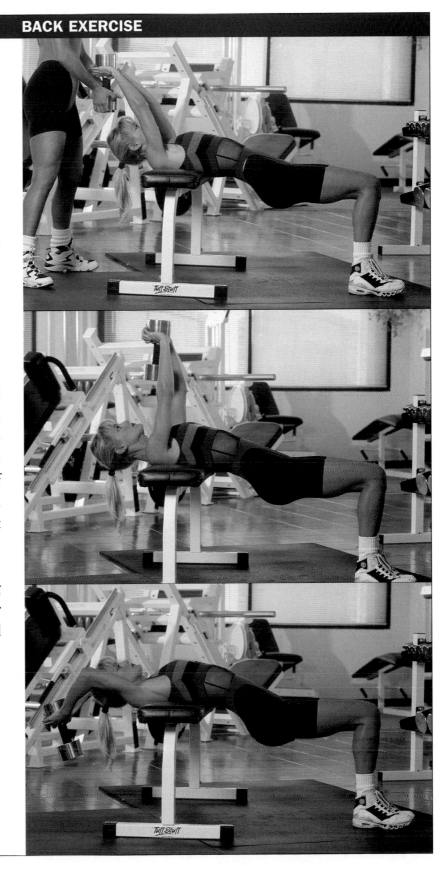

**BACK EXERCISE**

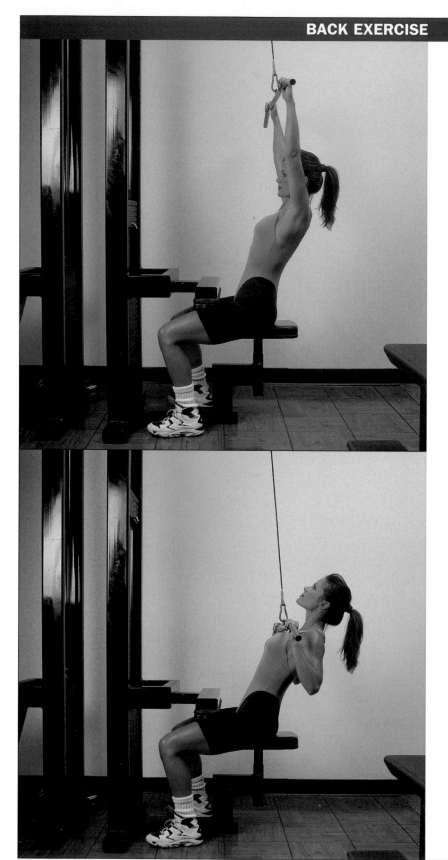

# Front pulldown

Take a shoulder-width grip on the bar. If you use an underhand grip, make sure it is less than shoulder-width.

Pull the bar down in front of your body to a position just below your shoulders. Lean back slightly. Do not let your chest "cave in."

Slowly return the bar to the starting position, and repeat the exercise for the suggested number of sets and repetitions.

**BACK EXERCISE**

# Seated cable row

Position yourself so that you sit facing the low-cable-pulley machine. Take a narrow grip, and lean forward.

While maintaining proper postural alignment (as pictured), pull your shoulders backward and arch your back slightly.

Pull the handle in toward your abdomen.

Return to the starting position, and repeat the exercise for the recommended number of sets and repetitions.

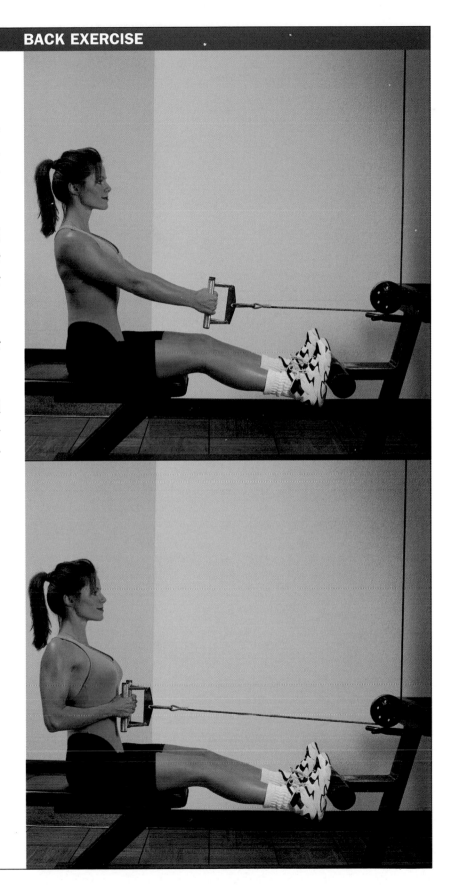

**BACK EXERCISE**

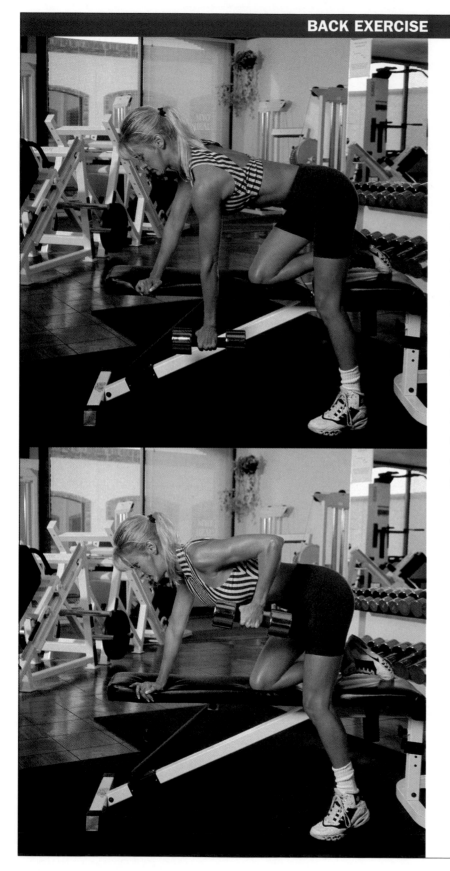

# One-arm dumbbell row

Place your left knee in the center of a flat exercise bench, with your opposite leg on the floor (your knee should be slightly bent, not locked).

Hold a dumbbell in your free hand.

Keeping your upper arm pressed close to your side, bend your elbow and bring the dumbbell up toward the side of your chest.

Lower the weight slowly to the starting position, and repeat the exercise for the required number of sets and repetitions.

**SHOULDER EXERCISE**

# Seated dumbbell shoulder press

Sit in a sturdy chair with both feet flat on the floor and your back firmly against the chair back.

Hold a dumbbell in each hand. Begin with the weights at shoulder level, with your palms facing forward.

Press the dumbbells upward, but without fully locking your elbow joints.

Slowly return to the starting position, and repeat the exercise for the recommended number of sets and repetitions.

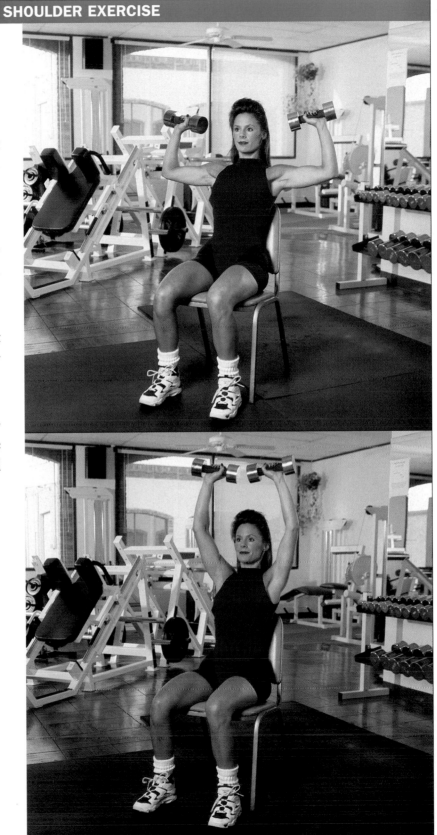

**SHOULDER EXERCISE**

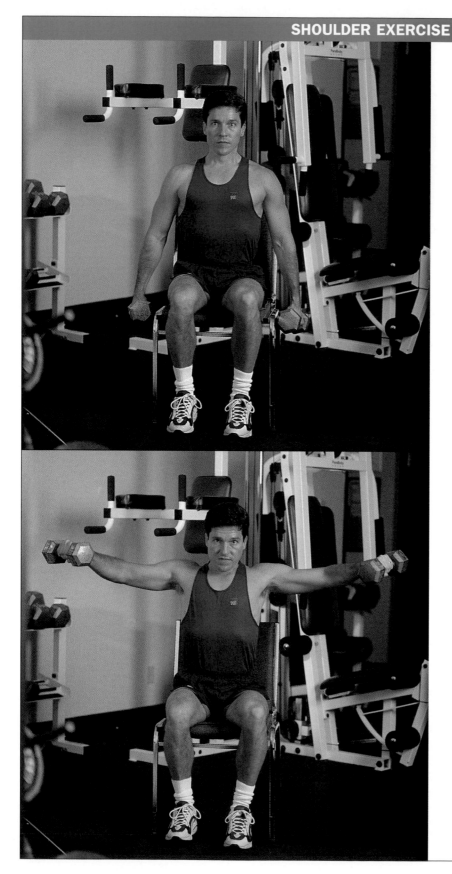

# Dumbbell lateral raise

Sit in a sturdy chair with both of your feet flat on the floor and your back pressed firmly against the chair back.

Grasp a dumbbell in each hand and hold the dumbbells at your sides, palms in.

Raise both elbows to at least shoulder height, maintaining about a 45-degree bend in your elbow joints throughout the exercise.

Slowly lower to the starting position, and repeat the exercise for the recommended number of sets and repetitions.

**SHOULDER EXERCISE**

# Upright row

Take an overhand grip on a barbell, placing your hands about shoulder-width apart. (Some people prefer a more narrow grip.)

Begin with the bar at thigh height. Keeping the bar close to your body, raise it to a shoulder-level position.

Lower slowly to the starting position, and repeat the exercise for the recommended number of sets and repetitions.

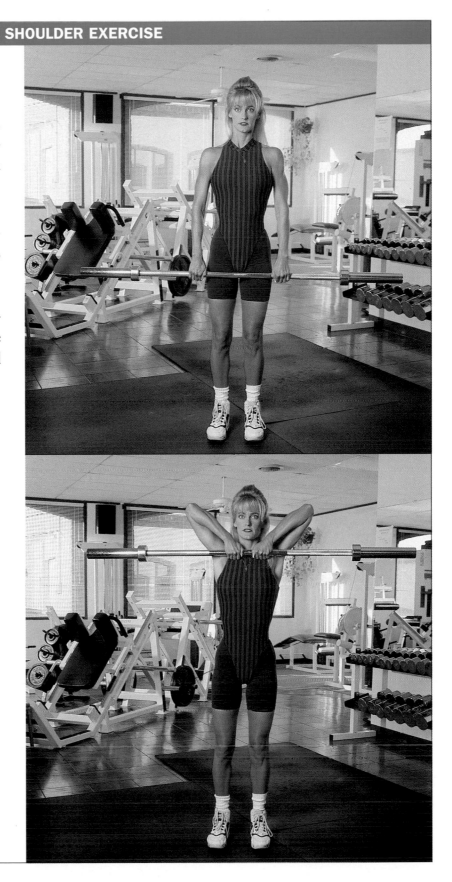

**SHOULDER EXERCISE**

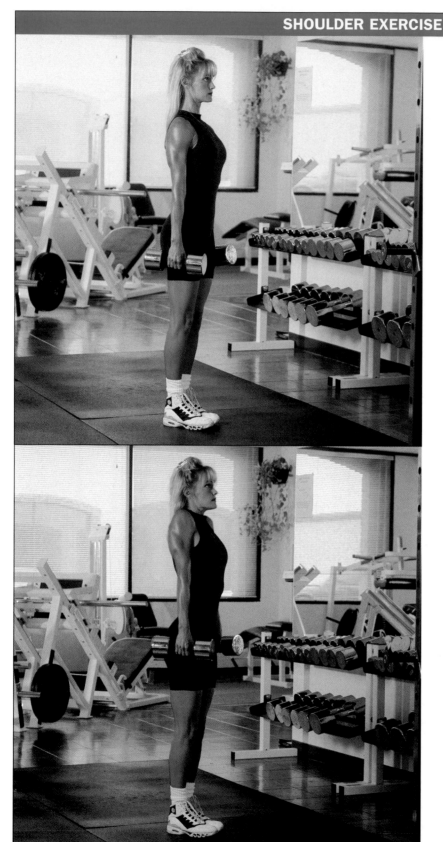

# Shrugs

Take a dumbbell in each hand and hold them at your sides.

Keeping your arms straight, raise your shoulders and trapezius muscles straight up, as high as you can, at least to a point just below your earlobes.

Hold the weight in the contracted position for a few moments.

Lower slowly to the starting position, and repeat the exercise for the recommended number of sets and repetitions. This exercise can also be performed with a barbell.

**TRICEPS EXERCISE**

# Triceps pressdown

*(only for exercisers without joint injuries)*

Face a high-cable-pulley machine, and stand with your feet slightly apart.

Grasp a short handle attached to the high pulley cable, palms facing down (overhand grip).

Hold your upper arms and elbows close to your body.

Maintaining this position, press the bar down toward the floor until your arms are fully extended and your elbows locked. In this position, tense your muscles.

Slowly return to the starting position, and repeat the exercise for the recommended number of sets and repetitions.

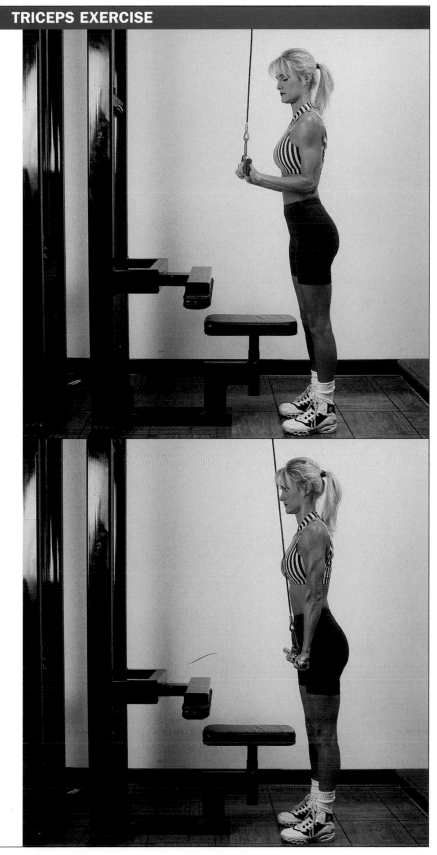

**TRICEPS EXERCISE**

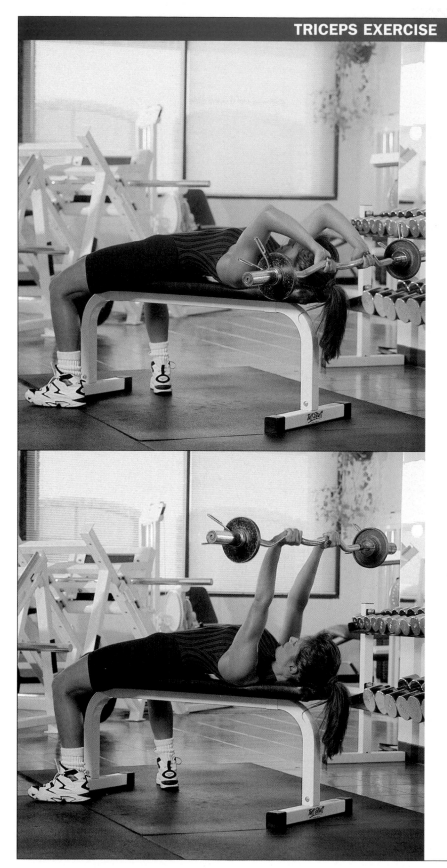

# Lying overhead triceps extension

Lie back on a flat exercise bench.

Grasp a barbell and hold it overhead with your arms extended. The angle of your arms should be slightly back.

Bend your elbows, letting the bar reach a position just behind your head. It is important to keep your arms stationary from the shoulder to the elbow throughout the exercise. Then press the bar back up, allowing it to travel in an arc back to the overhead position.

Slowly return to the starting position, and repeat the exercise for the recommended number of sets and repetitions.

**TRICEPS EXERCISE**

# Triceps kickback

Place your knee in the center of a flat exercise bench, with your opposite leg on the floor (knee joint unlocked). The arm that is opposite the leg on the floor should support you on the bench (see photograph).

Hold a dumbbell with your free hand.

Keeping your upper arm pressed close to your side, extend your arm straight out behind you. Keep your elbow as high as you can.

Flex at the elbow, bringing the weight toward the side of your chest. Then press your arm back out to the extended position.

Repeat the exercise for the recommended number of sets and repetitions.

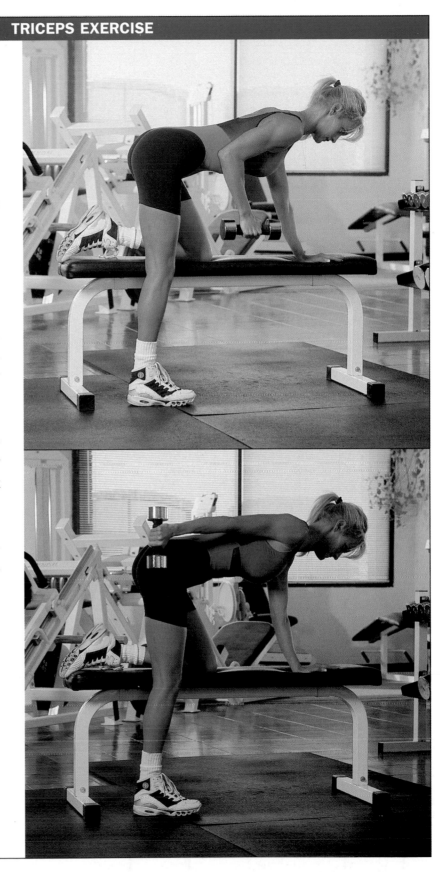

**TRICEPS EXERCISE**

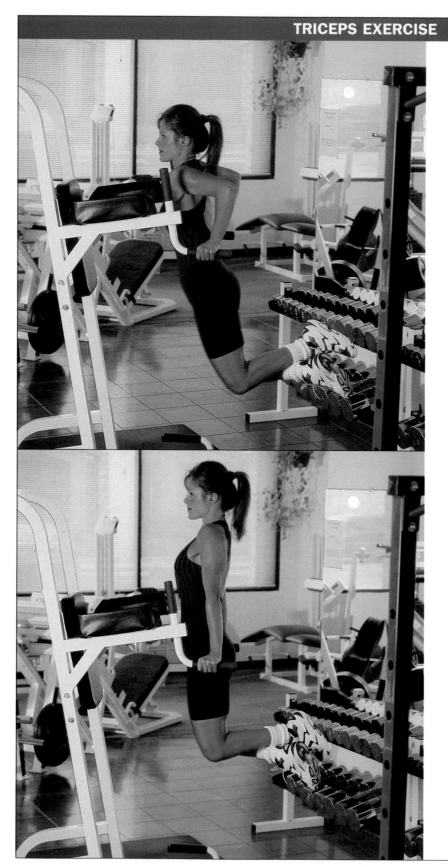

# Dips

To do the dip, grasp two parallel bars with your palms inward. Then push yourself up to a straight-arm position above the bars.

Bending your arms, lower your body slowly, as deeply as you can (but not below shoulder-level). Then straighten your arms and press your body back up.

Repeat the exercise for as many repetitions as you can.

**BICEPS EXERCISE**

# Barbell curl

Take an underhand grip on the barbell.

Begin the exercise with the barbell resting at upper-thigh level.

Flex your elbows, and bring the barbell up in an arc toward your chest. Tense your biceps at the top of the movement. Be sure to keep your upper arms close to your body.

Repeat the exercise for the recommended number of sets and repetitions. This exercise may also be performed with dumbbells.

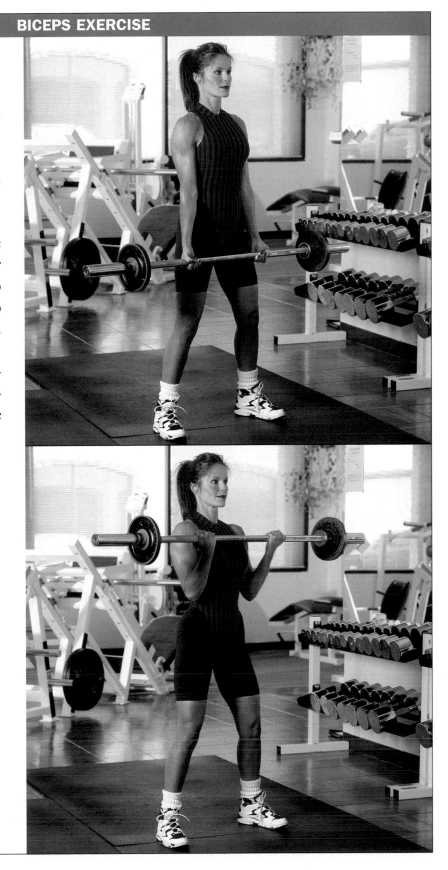

## BICEPS EXERCISE

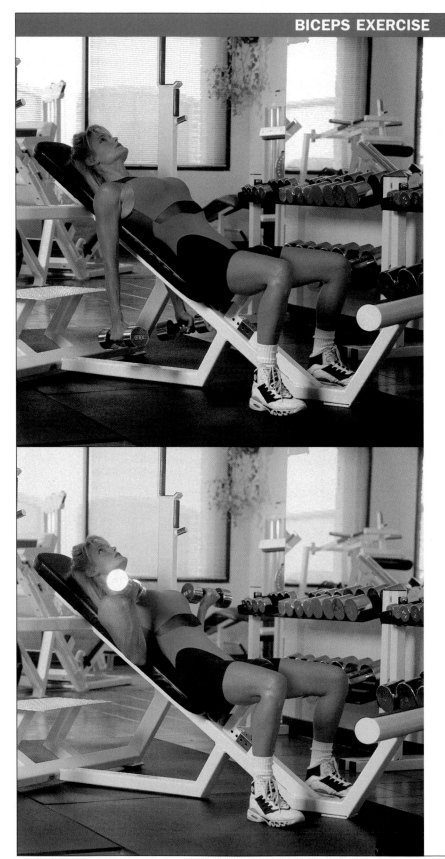

# Incline biceps curl

Sit back on the incline bench that has been set at a 45-degree angle. Your back should be flat against the bench, with your feet flat on the floor.

Take a dumbbell in each hand, palms facing in and arms extended downward. Your arms will be slightly behind your body.

Flex your elbows, curling dumbbells upward in an arc toward your shoulders. While curling upward, slowly turn the dumbbells outward.

Slowly return to the starting position, and repeat the exercise for the recommended number of sets and repetitions.

# Concentration curl

While seated on an exercise bench, take a dumbbell in one hand and rest your elbow against the inside of your thigh, as pictured. Your arm should be straight.

Lift the weight upward in an arc toward your shoulders and squeeze your biceps at the top of the movement.

Lower the weight slowly, and repeat the exercise for the recommended number of sets and repetitions.

Repeat the exercise with the other arm.

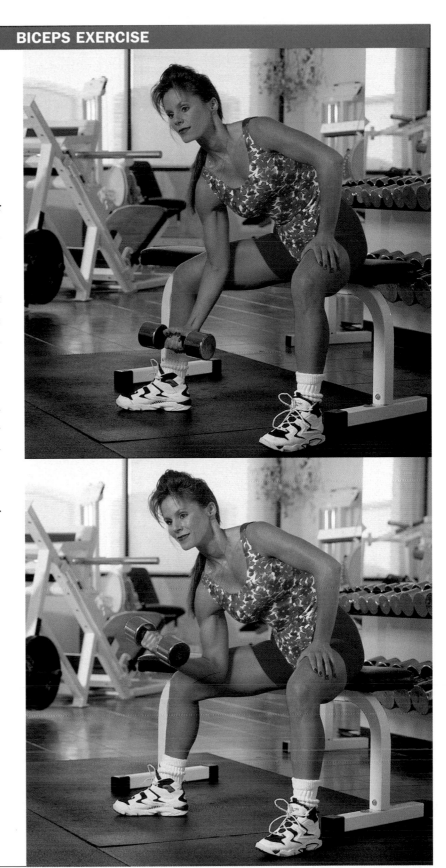

**BICEPS EXERCISE**

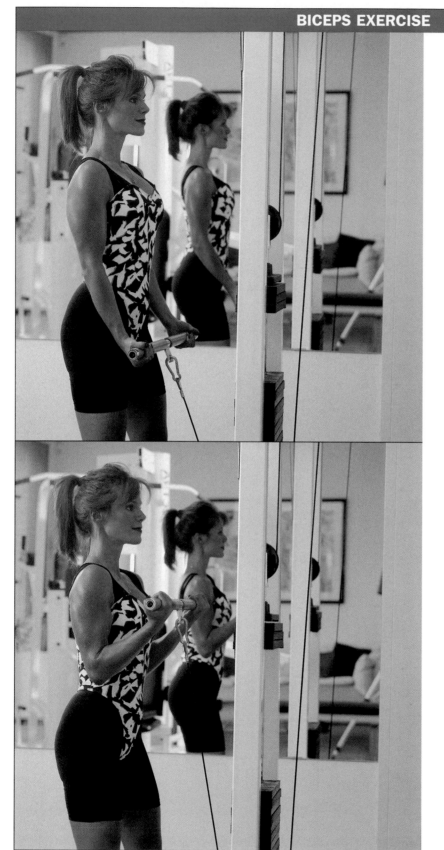

# Cable curls

Attach a short bar to the high pulley apparatus, and select a weight with which you can do 12 to 15 repetitions with some intensity of effort.

Take an underhand grip on the bar.

Begin the exercise with your arms extended down.

Flex your elbow joints, and curl upward until the bar reaches your chest. Keep your upper arms close to your sides.

Lower the weight slowly, and repeat the exercise for the recommended number of sets and repetitions.

**ABDOMINAL EXERCISE**

# Body crunch

Lie on your back on the floor with your knees bent and your arms placed behind your head as shown.

Contract your abdominal muscles, and lift your head, neck, shoulders, and upper back off the floor. Use the strength of your abdominals to perform this movement, not your lower back muscles.

Then lower to the starting position (shoulders off the floor), controlling the downward movement with your abdominal muscles.

Repeat the exercise for the recommended number of sets and repetitions.

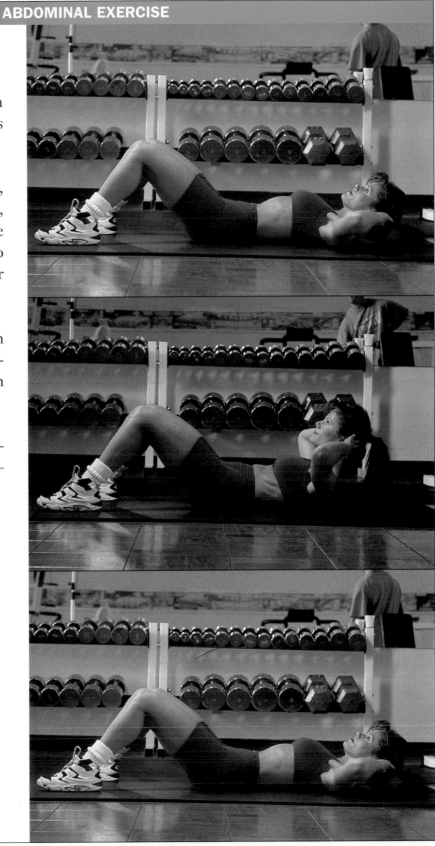

**ABDOMINAL EXERCISE**

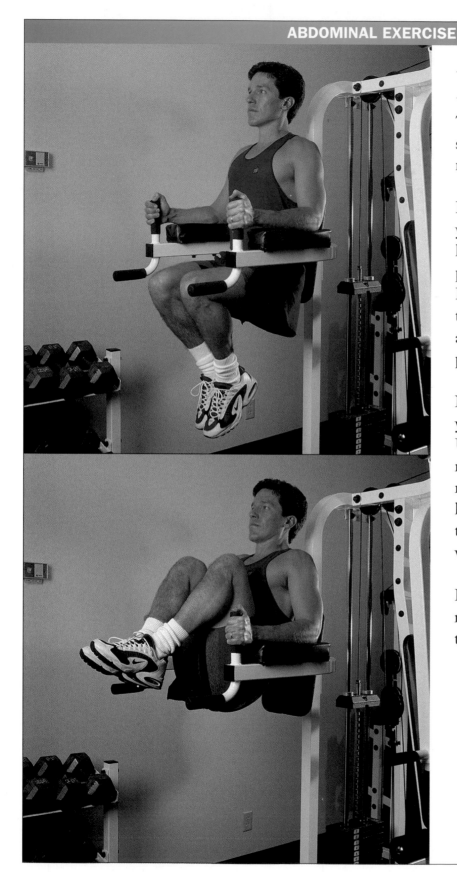

# Knee raise

This exercise is performed on a special apparatus designed for this movement.

Face forward as pictured, and hoist yourself up between the two parallel bars. Support yourself in this position with your legs straight. Bend your knees and pull your thighs upward so that they are parallel to the floor. This is the starting position.

Next, crunch your thighs toward your midsection as far as possible. Use the strength of your abdominals as you perform the exercise, not your lower back muscles. Then lower to the starting position, controlling the downward movement with your abdominal muscles.

Repeat the exercise for the recommended number of sets and repetitions.

**ABDOMINAL EXERCISE**

# Side crunch

Lie on your back on an exercise mat or the floor.

Bend your knees and cross one knee over the other, as pictured.

Place one hand behind your head; the other, extended out to your side.

Contract your abdominal muscles, and lift your head, neck, shoulders, and upper back off the floor.

Twist slightly to one side so that your bent elbow nearly meets the bent knee. Use the strength of your abdominals to perform this movement, not your lower back muscles. Then lower to the starting position (shoulders off the floor), controlling the downward movement with your abdominal muscles.

Repeat the exercise for the recommended number of sets and repetitions. Then repeat the exercise on the other side.

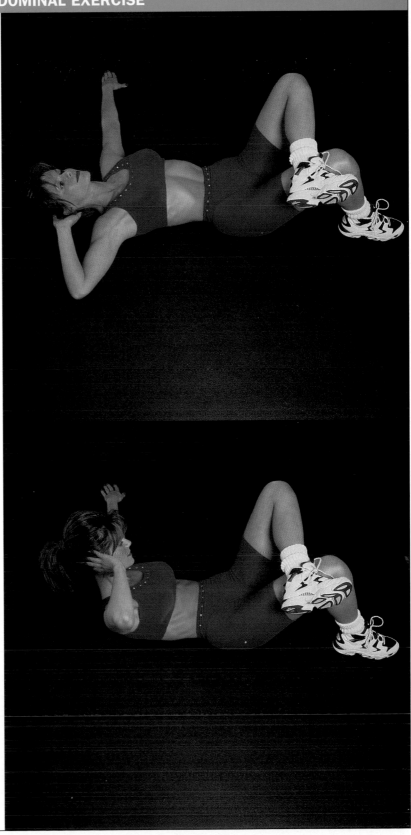

**ABDOMINAL EXERCISE**

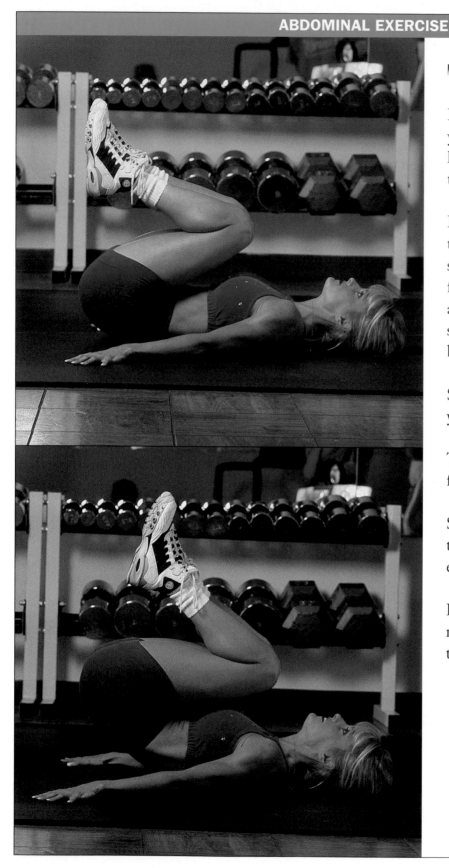

# Trunk raise

Lie on a mat or flat bench. Steady yourself by pressing your arms and hands on the mat or bench, as pictured.

Bend your knees and start pulling them toward your chest. Your knees should be bent with your thighs flexed at the hips so that your knees are over your torso. Your buttocks should not be touching the floor or bench. This is the starting position.

Shorten your torso by bringing your hips toward your head.

Tense your abdominal muscles forcefully.

Slowly return to the starting position, but without your buttocks ever touching the floor or bench.

Repeat the exercise for the recommended number of sets and repetitions.

**LOWER LEG EXERCISE**

# Standing calf raise

Stand with the ball of your foot on a block of wood or other elevated platform. Your other foot should be comfortably crossed behind your supporting leg. For support, hold onto a piece of equipment, stair rail, or other stationary item.

With your hand alongside your supporting (standing) leg, hold a dumbbell at your side, as pictured. Rise up on the ball of your foot as far as you can. Then lower your heel as deeply as possible, getting a good stretch.

Return to the starting position, and repeat the exercise for the recommended number of repetitions.

This exercise may be performed by pressing upward with the balls of both feet and without using weights, as pictured.

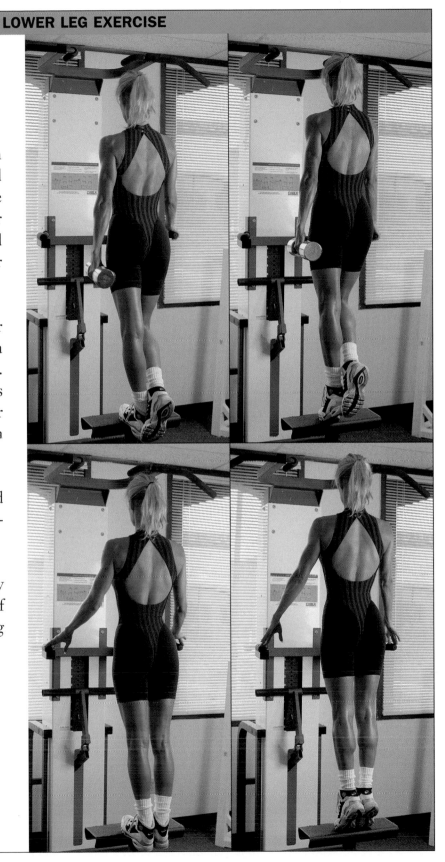

**LOWER LEG EXERCISE**

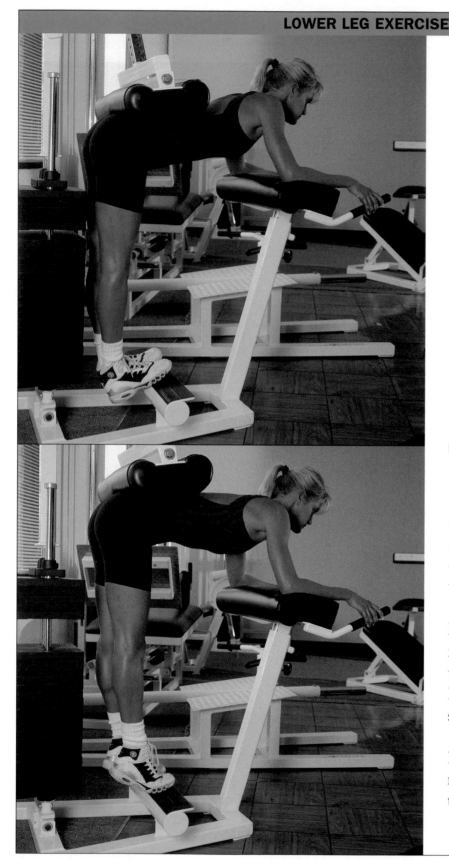

# Donkey calf raise

Position yourself in a donkey calf raise machine, as pictured. The pad should be resting on your lower back.

Support your upper torso by leaning on the backs of your forearms. Keep your back flat. Slowly lower your heels as far down as you can, getting a good stretch.

Return to the starting position, and repeat the exercise for the recommended number of repetitions.

# Seated calf raise

*This exercise is not pictured.*
Sit in the seated calf machine so that your legs are bent at a 90-degree angle. Make sure the pad fits evenly across your knees to distribute the load properly.

Press the weight upward by pushing against the pad across your thighs with the balls of your feel. Raise your heels up as high as possible. Then lower deeply.

Repeat the exercise for the recommended number of sets and repetitions.

# Chapter 18
## *Physique-Perfect Routines*

You have 30 days to a bathing suit-ready body. I'm sure you want to make the most of your time to get there. That's why the exercise routines on the Swimsuit Lean program are designed to target and tone the areas of the body most visible in a bathing suit—the midriff, thighs and hips, and upper body. Naturally you want those body parts to look the best they can when you're on the beach, at the pool, or on the deck of a cruise ship.

The exercise routines for Swimsuit Lean are not meant to "spot-reduce" areas with excess fat deposits, however. Spot-reduction attempts to use localized exercises to burn off fat in a certain area of the body. Yet to date no study has proved that such exercises can truly spot-reduce fat. However, there is some evidence suggesting that abdominal fat is burned more rapidly in response to exercise than fat from other areas of the body. I'll address that research later in this chapter.

What localized exercise *will* do is firm the muscle underneath the fat and make certain body parts look more defined. Aerobic exercise will help you burn fat from all areas of your body.

## How to Use the Swimsuit Lean Strength Training Routines

On your Swimsuit Lean strength training routine, you'll use either free weights or exercise machines. Free weights (exercises involving dumbbells and barbells) allow your joints to move freely through their full

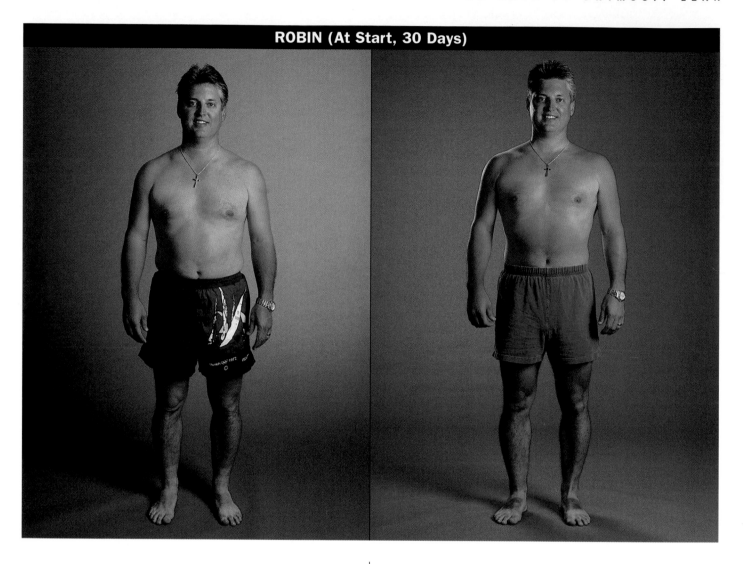

**ROBIN (At Start, 30 Days)**

range of motion. Machines move your body through a pre-set path and may not fit all body proportions the same way. However, machines are often easier for beginners to use. Both free weights and machines will help you achieve your Swimsuit Lean toning and strengthening goals

There are two basic, full-body strength training routines you can use on the Swimsuit Lean program—one for home (if you like to exercise at home), the other for the gym. Designed to be performed only twice a week, both routines are geared toward strengthening and firming the entire body. They are shown in Table 18-1 and Table 18-2 (see Chapter 17 for exercise instructions).

# Specialization Routines

The Swimsuit Lean program includes specialization routines you can perform in addition to your basic routine. Say your abs need extra attention. Then you would choose the abdominal specialization routine to help you "spot-shape" your midriff. Or if your thighs are trouble spots, try the thigh specialization routine. Whatever your goal, you can shape, firm, and strengthen these body parts through consistent training, dedicated effort, and adherence to my recommended eating program. Let's take a closer look at what you can do to trim and tone specific areas of your body.

## TABLE 18-1
# *Two-Day Basic Full-Body Routine for the Gym

| MUSCLE GROUPS | EXERCISE | SETS/REPETITIONS |
|---|---|---|
| Thighs/Buttocks | Leg press | 2 sets of 15 reps |
| | Leg extension (optional) | 2 sets of 15 reps |
| | Leg curl | 2 sets of 15 reps |
| Back | Seated row | 2 sets of 15 reps |
| | Front pulldown | 2 sets of 15 reps |
| Chest | Bench press (barbell or dumbbells) | 2 sets of 15 reps |
| | Dumbbell flys | 2 sets of 15 reps |
| Shoulders | Lateral raise (machine or dumbbells) | 2 sets of 15 reps |
| | Upright row (cable, barbell, or dumbbells) | 2 sets of 15 reps |
| Triceps | Dips or pushdowns | 2 sets of 15 reps |
| | Lying extensions (cable, barbell, or dumbbells) | 2 sets of 15 reps |
| Biceps | Standing barbell or dumbbell curl | 2 sets of 15 reps |
| | Concentration curl | 2 sets of 15 reps |
| Abdominals | Body crunch (machine or body weight) | 2 sets of 15 reps |
| Calves | Calf raise (donkey or seated) | 2 sets of 15 reps |

\* Be sure to warm up with 5 minutes of mild aerobics. I also advise performing a very light warm-up set before each exercise. This exercise routine shows working sets only.

## TABLE 18-2
# *Two-Day Basic Full-Body Routine for the Home

| MUSCLE GROUPS | EXERCISE | SETS/REPETITIONS |
|---|---|---|
| Thighs/Buttocks | Lunge | 2 sets of 15 reps |
| | Squats | 2 sets of 25 reps |
| Back | One-arm dumbbell row | 2 sets of 15 reps |
| | Dumbbell pullovers | 2 sets of 15 reps |
| Chest | Dumbbell bench press | 2 sets of 15 reps |
| | Dumbbell flys | 2 sets of 15 reps |
| Shoulders | Dumbbell lateral raise | 2 sets of 15 reps |
| Triceps | Lying triceps extensions | 2 sets of 15 reps |
| | Triceps kickbacks | 2 sets of 15 reps |
| Biceps | Standing barbell or dumbbell curl | 2 sets of 15 reps |
| Abdominals | Body crunch (body weight) | 2 sets of 25 reps |
| Calves | Standing calf raise | 2 sets of 15 reps |

\* Be sure to warm up with 5 minutes of mild aerobics. I also advise performing a very light warm-up set before each exercise. This exercise routine shows working sets only.

# Flatten and Firm Your Midriff

The four sets of muscles that make up your middle help you do everything from standing up to bending over. If you've ever had a lower back problem, you know that one of the most important steps in rehabilitation is to strengthen your abs. They serve an important purpose in protecting your spine. Unfortunately though, too many people carry excess fat around their waist—often the result of high-fat diets, on-again/off-again dieting, and lack of exercise.

"My middle has always been heavy—so much so that people would often mistake me for being pregnant, even when I wasn't!" one of our Swimsuit Lean participants told me. "The program has helped me reduce this area considerably. I look toned instead of flabby, and I'm getting more compliments than ever from my husband."

In addition to appearance problems, too much abdominal fat is a health hazard. Some examples:

## BLOOD SUGAR METABOLISM PROBLEMS

Fat cells in the abdomen tend to be larger than those in other parts of the body. This enlargement reduces the number of insulin receptors on the outer surface of cells. Under normal conditions, these receptors act like tiny doorbells. When insulin arrives on the doorstep of the cell, it "rings" the receptor doorbells, and the cell opens up to let glucose (blood sugar) come in. But with fewer receptors, the cells can't properly utilize glucose. This malfunction in turn causes glucose levels to rise. In response, the pancreas secretes more of the hormone insulin. Blood sugar metabolism can get out of whack, and full-blown dia-

betes can erupt. Excess weight around the waist is thus a risk factor for diabetes.[1]

## ENDOMETRIAL CANCER

Women whose body fat is distributed around and above the waist run a high risk of developing endometrial cancer, one of the most common cancers that afflict women. It usually occurs after menopause, and if detected early, it's almost always curable. Scientists speculate that one reason for the risk is because women with more abdominal fat have higher levels of the female hormone estrogen, which can set the stage for endometrial cancer.[2]

In a study of 40 women newly diagnosed with endometrial cancer and 40 controls matched for age, weight, and height, researchers found that the risk for this type of cancer increased as upper-body fat distribution increased. This finding led the researchers to conclude that upper-body fat distribution is a risk factor for endometrial cancer. Thus, by scaling down your upper-body fat, you scale down your risk for endometrial cancer, too.[3]

## HEART DISEASE

Excess upper-body and abdominal fat is also a risk for heart disease. Research has shown that upper-body-obesity results in unhealthy cholesterol profiles, high triglycerides (blood fats), and high blood pressure—which can all spell heart trouble.[4]

A lot of men with pot bellies will say they aren't really fat. Reason? Because their bellies are rock hard to the touch. But all this means is that excess fat in their abdominal cavity is pushing against their abdominal muscles and stretching them so tightly that their bellies do feel hard. So, guys, take heed: Weight around the middle is very health-risky. Fortunately, though, the risks don't necessarily apply to you if you exercise regularly and follow a healthy diet.[5]

# Exercise to the Rescue

From a cosmetic viewpoint, abs are a focal point. Having a toned, tight midriff as opposed to a spare tire helps you look trimmer. Fortunately, abdominal fat is easier to shed than fat from other parts of the body such as the thighs and hips where fat cells tend to be more stubborn. The reason has to do with enzymes, which split fat into small pieces so it can move in and out of storage. It just so happens that enzymes in abdominal fat tissue are among the most active anywhere in the body's fat depots—so active that fat moves easily out of abdominal storage sites, particularly in response to exercise. In other words, more fat is lost first from your waist as a result of exercise.[6]

Some recent scientific experiments have shed some light on just how exercise affects abdominal fat:

At the Washington University School of Medicine in St. Louis, researchers assigned a group of men and women, aged 60 to 70, to a nine to twelve-month exercise program of walking or jogging. On average, the participants worked out 45 minutes several times a week—which is what I recommend on the Swimsuit Lean program. Furthermore, they exercised at 80 percent of their maximum heart rate, an intensity level geared for fat-burning and cardiovascular conditioning. By the end of the study, all the participants had lost weight. But the most significant finding was this: Most of the lost weight was trimmed from the abdominal area.[7]

If walking and jogging are good waist-slimmers, what about strength training? Researchers at the University of Alabama looked into this.

They put 14 healthy older women on a total-body strength-training program to see if this form of exercise would reduce intra-abdominal fat (fat inside the abdominal cavity rather than just under the skin). Before and after the study, the researchers measured the women's body composition using CT scans and underwater weight, two highly accurate measurement methods. The women worked out three times a week for 16 weeks. By the end of the experiment, there were significant reductions in intra-abdominal fat—so significant, in fact, that the researchers felt these positive changes could be an important factor in overcoming the health risks associated with excess abdominal fat, especially as we age.[8]

The lesson in these studies is that that a consistent program of aerobic exercise *and* strength training can help whittle away abdominal fat—and keep you healthier as a result.

## *The Swimsuit Lean*
## Mid-Section
## Specialization Routine

Shown in Table 18-3 is a specialization routine for the abs. Perform it at least twice a week on non-consecutive days, and make sure to do fat-burning aerobic exercise as recommended. As long as you continue your aerobics and eating program, your abs will "waist away" in no time at all!

# Firm Up Your
# Bottom Line

Your thigh and hips muscles are used daily—to walk, stand up, and sit down. Because of their near-constant use, they can be slow in responding to exercise. What's more, the fat in these regions is difficult to mobilize and burn in response to exercise, especially in women. One main reason has to do with childbearing. Women need that fat for menstruation, pregnancy, and lactation. Only during lactation does the body willingly give up fat cells on the lower body—to support the energy needs of the nursing baby.

Still, with intensity of effort, the Swimsuit Lean eating program, and regular aerobic exercise, you can sculpt your legs and hips to the level of shape and strength you desire.

# Lower Body Fat and Your Health

The health consequences of excess lower body fat are not as severe as those related to abdominal fat. One risk of lower body fat, however, is osteoarthritis, a disabling joint disease that affects millions of people. In osteoarthritis, there's a gradual breakdown of cartilage (a soft tissue that pads the ends of bones at joints), and sometimes bone, from overuse, stress on the joints, and unrepaired injury. When enough cartilage has worn away, the surfaces of bones start grinding together, causing pain and stiffness. Progressive and often crippling, osteoarthritis affects the knees, spine, hips, feet, and other body parts.

A critical risk factor for osteoarthritis is excess weight, which burdens the joints and aggravates the course of their wear and tear. Keeping your weight under control through proper diet and exercise is one way to prevent osteoarthritis.

If you do have osteoarthritis, one way that may help manage it naturally is with a supplement called Cosamin. This supplement is a mixture of chondroitin sulfates, which are found naturally in cartilage, and glucosamine, a sugar molecule manufactured by cartilage cells from glucose and the amino acid, glutamine.

## *The Swimsuit Lean*
# Thigh and Hip Specialization Routine

Shown in Table 18-4 is a specialization routine for the hips and thighs. You may perform it twice a week on non-consecutive days, and make sure to do fat-burning aerobic exercise as recommended. Stick to your aerobics and eating program, and your bottom line will start looking better very soon!

# A Tapered, Toned Upper Body

I suspect that most men are interested in having an impressive upper body—broad shoulders and a tapered, V-shaped upper back. But women can benefit from the same look. By developing your shoulders, back, and chest more fully, you can offset wide hips or a thick waist, creating a more balanced figure. Not only that, your posture improves when upper body muscles are toned.

Prior to starting the Swimsuit Lean program, Angel B.'s number-one goal was to strengthen and develop her upper body, particularly her arms, back, and chest. Angel, who had never worked out with weights before, started a strength training program of two workouts a week, as recommended on the program. "Before long, my husband noticed that I could move furniture without any problem," she said. "And I noticed that my back and arms are stronger when I'm holding my

| TABLE 18-3 |
|:---:|
| ***Mid-Section Specialization Routine\**** |

| EXERCISE | SETS/REPETITIONS |
|---|---|
| Trunk raise | 1 to 2 sets of 15 to 25 reps |
| Side crunch | 1 to 2 sets of 15 to 25 reps |
| Knee-raise | 1 to 2 sets of 15 to 25 reps |

*If your mid-section needs extra attention, perform this routine in addition to one of the basic full-body routines. These abdominal exercises should be performed following the body crunch exercise in either the full-body gym routine or the full-body home routine.

| TABLE 18-4 |
|:---:|
| ***Thigh and Hip Specialization Routine\**** |

| EXERCISE | SETS/REPETITIONS |
|---|---|
| Hack squat | 2 sets of 12 to 15 reps |
| Straight leg deadlift | 2 sets of 12 to 15 reps |
| Lunge | 2 sets of 12 to 15 reps |

*If your hips and thighs need extra attention, perform this routine in place of the hip and thigh exercises found in either of the basic full-body routines. Also, if your hips and thighs are lagging in development, give them priority when you work out. In other words, exercise them first in your routine when your energy levels are at their highest, thus giving these body parts full attention. I also suggest that you gradually work up to performing additional repetitions and sets on body parts that need additional shape-up work.

| TABLE 18-5 |
|:---:|
| ***Upper Body Specialization Routine\**** |

| MUSCLE GROUPS | EXERCISE | SETS/REPETITIONS |
|---|---|---|
| Upper back | Chins | As many as you can |
| Chest | Dumbbell bench press or barbell bench press | 2 sets of 12 to 15 reps |
| Shoulders | Seated dumbbell shoulder press and lateral press if not already incorporated in your program | 2 sets of 12 to 15 reps |
|  | Shrugs | As many as you can |

*If your upper body (shoulders, chest, and back) needs extra attention, perform this routine in place of the upper back, chest, and shoulder exercises in either of the basic full-body routines. Also, if your upper body is lagging in development, give it priority when you work out. In other words, exercise it first in your routine when your energy levels are at their highest, thus giving these body parts full attention. I also suggest that you gradually work up to performing additional repetitions and sets on body parts that need additional shape-up work.

grandchild. I just feel so much stronger. Plus, I'm leaner around my ribcage, I've got less flab on my arms, and my posture is taller and straighter."

There are benefits for everyone in having a stronger, shapelier upper body. A strong upper body protects you against potential athletic injuries, particularly in your shoulders and back. Even everyday aches and pains, such as low back problems, caused by muscular weakness, can be alleviated by getting stronger.

As Angel learned, the ability to accomplish such day-to-day tasks is another benefit of having a strong, well-developed upper body. And if you're an athlete, you'll have the stamina and power to throw farther, swing harder, hit more powerfully.

Shown in Table 18-5 is the Swimsuit Lean specialization routine for the upper body. Be sure to perform fat-burning aerobic exercise as recommended.

# Swimsuit Lean Maintenance

# Chapter 19
## The New You, Inside and Out

In April 1996, news agencies across the country reported the death of National League baseball umpire John McSherry, whose weight had ballooned to 400 pounds. He suffered a heart attack, collapsed behind home plate, and died about an hour later.

Not long afterward, baseball officials gave another umpire, Eric Gregg, a leave of absence so he could trim down his 325-pound frame. Gregg was quoted in wire reports as saying: "In light of recent events, I feel this is the right time to take a serious look at my weight and conditioning. My goal is to be a major-league umpire for many years to come, and to accomplish that I need to take a closer look at my overall health."[1]

Being overweight is clearly a life-and-death matter. About 300,000 lives are lost each year due to overweight and obesity. In fact, weight-related illnesses are the second leading cause of death* in the United States.[2]

What are those illnesses? Let's take a closer look.

## Heart Disease

Without a doubt, the most serious is heart disease, the leading killer of men and women in the United States. What's more, it costs business approximately $3 billion a year in lost workdays.[3]

Being overweight increases the risk factors for heart disease, particularly high blood pressure, high triglycerides (a type of blood fat), and

* Smoking is the leading cause of death among Americans, resulting in an estimated 500,000 deaths annually.

high blood cholesterol (obese people tend to have lower levels of the "good" HDL cholesterol and high levels of the "bad" LDL cholesterol).

Like rust building up inside a pipe, excess saturated fat in the diet can cause an accumulation of cholesterol inside the walls of your arteries, forming a by-product called plaque that clogs the arteries. This build-up is part of a disease called atherosclerosis, a progressive condition that can begin in childhood and can cause killer complications such as heart attacks and stroke in adulthood.

God gave us a logical mind to form logical conclusions. Thus, when it comes to heart disease, it's this simple: What you put in your mouth is critical to your health. Research has shown us that the prevention of heart disease through proper diet and exercise is a real possibility for many people. For those who already suffer from heart disease or are high-risk candidates, research further shows that proper diet and exercise may slow down—in some cases possibly reverse—some of the effects of the disease.

One reason has to do with fat loss. When you lose body fat, your cholesterol level drops. Based on the results of more than 70 scientific studies, researchers have concluded that for every five pounds you lose, your total cholesterol drops by 7 points, LDL cholesterol by 3 points, and triglycerides by 14 points. Furthermore, HDL cholesterol goes up by 1 point. These favorable changes in blood fats all cut your chances of getting heart disease.[4]

Fiber is a key factor in heart disease protection too. Fiber-rich foods like whole grain cereals, oat bran, wheat bran, corn, barley, and legumes clean out more than your digestive tract. Fiber also roots out harmful levels of LDL cholesterol to ultimately protect you from heart disease. The best way to increase the fiber in your diet is to increase the amount of grains, beans, and vegetables you eat.

Sometime soon, you might want to have a blood test to see if your cholesterol and triglycerides have dropped as a result of your low-fat eating, active lifestyle, and lost fat. When those levels decline, your heart gets in better shape—as long as you stay in shape. By contrast, regaining weight increases dangerous cholesterol levels in your blood. This results in a build-up of fat deposits around the heart and in the walls of your arteries.[5]

# High Blood Pressure

Then there's the issue of high blood pressure. High blood pressure is a symptom-less disease, but one so serious that it has been dubbed "the silent killer." More than 60 million Americans have it, although almost half of them don't even know it. There are usually no early warning signals. High blood pressure slowly works its evil, causing long-term damage to your heart, blood vessels, and kidneys. Even with a diagnosis of mild high blood pressure, you have double the risk of heart attack as does a person with normal blood pressure. The best way to detect this silent killer is to have your blood pressure taken regularly.

Whatever its cause, high blood pressure is one of the most treatable—and one of the most preventable—of all killer diseases. The mainstay of treatment for high blood pressure has traditionally been prescription medication. Evidence continues to mount, however, that diets rich in blood-pressure lowering calcium, potassium, magnesium, and other nutrients, may be just as effective, but without the side effects of drugs.[6]

# Stroke

Stroke is the lightning bolt of circulatory diseases—striking without much warning and leaving survivors and their families in a state of shock. The third leading cause of death in the United States, stroke is a disabler and a killer. Each year, more than 500,000 Americans suffer stroke. About one-fourth of them die; the rest may be permanently disabled due to neurological damage that cannot be repaired or reversed.[7]

Stroke is an illness that often stems from other diseases—high blood pressure, heart disease, diabetes, and high cholesterol. If these can be prevented, stroke can be prevented, too.

One of the best ways to do that: healthy nutrition. Changing to a diet rich in natural, unrefined starchy and fibrous carbohydrates definitely reduces your chances of stroke. One reason is that these foods are high in potassium, magnesium, vitamin C, and other anti-stroke nutrients. As a part of the well-known Framingham Study, researchers tracked 832 men, ages 45 to 65, for 20 years. As their intake of fruit and vegetables increased, their risk of stroke dropped. The researchers concluded that eating more fruits and vegetables may protect against the development of stroke in men. And the same may be true in women.[8]

# Cancer

Cancer is a complex disease, yet new links between cancer and diet are being discovered all the time. Is cancer related to overweight and obesity? The American Cancer Society thinks so. The society reports that deaths from cancer increase in people who are overweight, especially women.

According to a study conducted by the society, overweight women have higher rates of endometrial, gallbladder, cervical, ovarian, and breast cancers. Furthermore, overweight men have higher rates of colon and prostate cancers.[9]

A healthy diet appears to be cancer-protective. Many types of cancers are rare in populations of people who eat lots of vegetables and whole grains. There may be several reasons for this: the high-fiber content of these foods, their higher concentration of antioxidants, and their phytochemical content.

# Diabetes

Another life-threatening disease is Type II (noninsulin dependent) diabetes, a blood sugar disorder in which the body's cells do not let in enough glucose for proper nourishment. Scientists estimate that 88 to 97 percent of all cases of Type II diabetes diagnosed in overweight people are directly related to their weight problem.[10] Both diet and exercise can help prevent and control Type II diabetes. According to scientific research, overweight diabetics who lost at least 15 pounds in a year lowered their blood sugar level by 15 percent—without having to take medication. Diabetics who lost 30 pounds reduced their blood sugar by 40 percent.[11]

# You Have a Choice

Fortunately, as umpire Eric Gregg did, you can do something about your health and prevent overweight-related illnesses. Clearly, today's chronic diseases are influenced greatly by diet, exercise, and other lifestyle factors (these are summarized in Table 19-1). That means that many of the risk

**TABLE 19-1**

## Diet and Lifestyle Factors Linked to Serious Disease

| DISEASE | RISK FACTOR |
| --- | --- |
| Coronary heart disease | Diets high in animal fat and cholesterol, obesity, smoking, lack of exercise |
| Type II diabetes | Obesity, low-fiber diets, diets high in processed foods |
| Cancer | Diets high in animal fat and low in fiber, antioxidants, and vegetables; smoking; lack of exercise |
| High blood pressure | Obesity, diets high in salt and animal fat, smoking, lack of exercise |
| Stroke | Obesity, diets high in salt and animal fat, smoking, lack of exercise |
| Osteoporosis | Diets low in calcium and vitamin D, lack of exercise |
| Gallbladder disease | Obesity |
| Osteoarthritis | Obesity |

factors for disease can be reduced or eliminated. How you live day-to-day affects your long-term health and quality of life.

Though his general health had always been good, Jerry M. had a few problems that could be managed by proper diet, namely sky-high cholesterol and triglycerides and borderline high blood pressure. "I was flirting with disaster," Jerry says. "But now, everything is within acceptable ranges. This should help maintain the good health I've always enjoyed."

From the moment you started the Swimsuit Lean program, your body began to change. Your body fat percentage headed down, while your lean muscle headed up. These are changes you can see.

But there are some changes you can't readily see—like an improved cholesterol profile, better-nourished cells, a faster-running metabolism, a more efficient cardiovascular system, to name just a few. By changing your diet and activity level for the better, you're improving your health and protecting your quality of life. And the Swimsuit Lean program, along with its maintenance program, is a step in the right direction.

# Chapter 20

## Ever-After Lean

*N*ow that you're swimsuit lean…what do you do next?

Stay that way—with my Swimsuit Lean maintenance program. If you have reached your goals after 30 days, here's all you have to do to stay lean:

1. Re-introduce all fruits (bananas, grapes, oranges, etc.) back into your weekly meal plans by eating two to three pieces of fruit daily.

2. If you desire, schedule one meal a week to eat anything you like. No foods are off bounds at this particular meal. But be reasonable; do not binge! A single meal of non-restricted eating is of little consequence in terms of fat loss and maintenance. It gives you an eating freedom that will prevent a total relapse into unhealthy, high-fat eating habits.

3. Once a day, you may substitute one serving of a refined, processed carbohydrate—for example, 1/2 cup of pasta, one bagel, or one slice of white bread—for your usual natural, unrefined carbohydrate.

4. As for exercise, continue to train with weights *at least* twice a week. Strive to increase your workout intensity.

5. Continue to perform aerobics *at least* three to four days a week. Again, strive to increase your exercise intensity. One of the most influential factors in staying lean is maintaining a regular exercise program.

6. Continue to monitor your body composition and weight every few weeks. If you find that your body fat percentage is climbing again, analyze your diet and course-correct if you're eating too many high-fat or refined, processed foods. Be sure to follow the Swimsuit Lean recommendations for exercise, too.

# If You Have More Body Fat to Lose

By the end of the 30-day period, you may still have more fat to lose and may not be ready for maintenance. If so, follow these recommendations:

1. Stay on the eating program at the caloric level you reached by the fourth week or use your optimal fueling formulas on page 39.

2. Continue to weight train at least twice a week.

3. Continue your aerobic exercise program, performing aerobics at least four to five times a week, as recommended on days 8 through 14 of the Swimsuit Lean program. Try to do those aerobic sessions at the best "fat-burning" times—before breakfast, after dinner in the evenings, and after strength training workouts.

4. Monitor your body composition weekly. This reading will help you make the proper adjustments. For example, let's say you plateau; you're not losing any more body fat. That being the case, you may need to boost your metabolism. There are several ways to do this. For example:

   ■ Increase the frequency and/or the duration of your aerobics.

   ■ Gradually add 100 more calories to your eating program while increasing your activity accordingly.

   ■ Up the intensity of your strength training workouts (lift heavier weights or increase the number of repetitions and workout more than twice a week).

   ■ Further restrict your intake of starchy carbohydrates in the evenings.

Most people who follow the Swimsuit Lean maintenance program make further progress. Angela S., for example, continued to "thin out in the middle," while enjoying the extra freedom of maintenance eating.

# Manage Stress to Help Keep Body Fat Off

Stress is your body's response to any physical, mental, or psychological demand. What many people don't realize is that stress can interfere with efforts to stay lean. During stress, the body tries to compensate physiologically by triggering the release of hormones that increase levels of blood sugar and blood fats. If stress continues without interruption, the body enters a state of exhaustion, which can ultimately result in disease. Stress management is thus an important factor in weight control and disease prevention.

One way to manage stress is through proper nutrition. A moderately high-protein diet, for example, provides all the essential amino acids necessary for cellular repair. The Swimsuit Lean meals are also high in certain nutrients easily depleted by stress, namely antioxidants and B-complex vitamins. Supplementing with vitamin E* (at least 400 IUs daily) is a good idea too, since this nutrient affords protection against stress.[1] By giving your body the nutritional resources it needs, you help insure yourself against stress.

Here are some additional stress-management pointers:

■ Do learn to slow down. The constant need to do more in less time causes enormous frustration for many people. That "swimming

*Check with your physician before using vitamin/mineral supplements.

upstream" feeling we all experience at times can be physically harmful.

■ Don't neglect nutrition, exercise, or sleep. A disruption in the balance of diet, exercise, and sleep allows stressors to do their damage on your body and mind.

■ Don't alter your living patterns too quickly. Because change is a stressor, significant changes in your life should be eased into slowly. Athletes always warm up before the game; your body, mind, and emotions also need a "warm up." For example, if you begin to rise one hour earlier in the morning, compensate by going to bed one hour earlier at night.

■ Don't overindulge; try to practice moderation. Excessive behavior disrupts the body's natural rhythm. Too much alcohol, for instance, will disrupt your immune system.

■ Don't expect too much from yourself. You're only human, so forgive yourself when you make a mistake. You'll enjoy life more—and people will enjoy you more—if you learn not to take too seriously those everyday ups and downs. Enjoy today.

# From Here to Lean

In contrast to most "diets," Swimsuit Lean is something you'll want to stay with indefinitely—in other words, this program is so effortless that you'll want it as part of your lifestyle from here on out.

Hopefully, you'll realize that the natural foods emphasized on this program are incredibly healthful for your body. Greens, grains, legumes, low-fat proteins, and other valuable foods are vital for keeping you well, not to mention lean! Who would want to give them up just because the 30 days are over?

Likewise, who would want to give up all the health and body-shaping benefits of regular exercise? Quite probably, you'll want to continue to eat and exercise this way—and be lean and healthy throughout the golden years of your life!

# Appendix

## A

### Recommended Products

**Vitamins:**
Beverly International Ultra 4 Vitamin/Mineral Formula™

**Minerals:**
Beverly International Ultra 4 Vitamin/Mineral Formula™

**Lipotropics:**
Parrillo Advanced Lipotropic Formula™

**Carbohydrate supplements:**
Parrillo ProCarb™

**Creatine monohydrate:**
Parrillo Creatine Monohydrate™

**Cosamin**

**Protein supplements:**
Parrillo Hi-Protein Powder,™ Vita-Herb Protein Powder, and Beverly International 100% Egg White Protein Powder

**Sports Nutrition Bar:**
Parrillo Supplement Bar

**MCT Oil:**
Parrillo CapTri®

**Longhorn Beef:**
To order, call or write
Springer Hill Ranch
P. O. Box 5121, Ovilla, Texas 75154
214-522-7812.

**Please note:** Parrillo supplements, as well as Cosamin, may be ordered by calling Lean Bodies at 1-800-697-LEAN.
For counseling call 972-380-LEAN

## B

### Recommended Reading

**Cliff Sheats' Lean Bodies: The Revolutionary Approach To Losing Body Fat By Increasing Calories** by Cliff Sheats and Maggie Greenwood-Robinson (The Summit Publishing Group, Warner Books, 1992, 1995).

**Cliff Sheats' Lean Bodies Cookbook** by Cliff Sheats and Linda Thornbrugh (The Summit Publishing Group, Warner Books, 1992, 1995).

**Cliff Sheats' Lean Bodies Total Fitness** by Cliff Sheats and Maggie Greenwood-Robinson (The Summit Publishing Group, 1996).

**High Performance Bodybuilding** by John Parrillo and Maggie Greenwood-Robinson (Perigee Books, 1993).

**John Parrillo's 50 Workout Secrets** by John Parrillo and Maggie Greenwood-Robinson (Perigee Books, 1994).

**Shape Training: The 8-Week Total Body Makeover** by Robert Kennedy and Maggie Greenwood-Robinson (Contemporary Books, 1996).

# References

A major portion of the information in this book comes from personal case studies with participants in the Swimsuit Lean program, medical research reports in both the popular and scientific publications, professional textbooks, and computer searches of medical databases of research abstracts.

## Chapter 1
**What to Expect in 30 Days**
1. Melvin H. Williams, Nutrition for Fitness and Sport, 2nd. ed. (Dubuque, Iowa: W. C. Brown, 1988), 252.

## Chapter 3
**Anti-Fat, Pro-Health Nutrients**
1. "Dietary Fiber Helps Some to Lose Weight," Better Nutrition for Today's Living 56 (October 1994): 34.
2. M.A. Gorman and C. Bowman, "Position of the American Dietetic Association: Health Implications of Dietary Fiber," Journal of the American Dietetic Association 93 (1993): 1446-1447.
3. Sharon Begley, "Beyond Vitamins," Newsweek, April 25, 1994, 44-49.
4. Ibid.
5. Ibid.
6. Mark J. Messina, "Dietary Phytoestrogens: Cancer Cause or Prevention?" The Soy Connection 3 (Fall 1994): 1-4.
7. Susan Kleiner, "Antioxidant Answers," The Physician and Sportsmedicine 24 (August 1996): 21-22.
8. G.P. Oakley, Jr., M.J. Adams, and C.M. Dickinson, "More Folic Acid for Everyone, Now," Journal of Nutrition 126 (March 1996): 751S-755S.
9. E. Jennings, "Folic Acid as a Cancer-Preventing Agent," Medical Hypotheses 45 (September 1995): 297-303.
10. R. Grio, R. Piacentino, G.L. Marchino, and R. Navone, "Antineoblastic Activity of Antioxidant Vitamins: The Role of Folic Acid in the Prevention of Cervical Dysplasia," Panminerva Medicine 35 (December 1993): 193-6.
11. Judy McBride, "How Sweet It Isn't," Agricultural News 39 (July 1991), 20-24.
12. R. R. Henry, P.A. Crapo, and A.W. Thorburn, "Current Issues in Fructose Metabolism," Annual Review of Nutrition 1991 11: 21-39; McBride, 20-24.
13. "Metabolic Effects of Fructose," Nutrition Research Newsletter 11 (April 1992), 51-52.
14. Susan M. Smith, "Sugar Substitutes May Play Positive Roles in Weight Loss," Environmental Nutrition 12 (March 1989): 1-2.
15. Ibid.
16. Associated Press, "Substitute for Fat Attacked as Unsafe," Evansville Courier, October 26, 1995, A10.

## Chapter 4
**Anti-Fat Supplements**
1. Reported in: General Nutrition Centers, Inc., "Formula for Success," Annual Report (1995): 1.
2. Frank Murray, "Athletes Have Increased Vitamin and Mineral Needs," Today's Living 21 (April 1990): 6.
3. G. I. Dragan, A. Vasiliu, E. Georgescu, and N. Eremia, "Studies Concerning Chronic and Acute Effects of L-carnitina in Elite Athletes," Physiologie 26 (April-June 1989): 111-129; G. I. Dragan, W. Wagner, and E. Ploesteanu, "Studies concerning the Ergogenic Value of Protein Supply and L-carnitine in Elite Junior Cyclists," Physiologie 25 (July-September 1988): 129-132.
4. W.W. Campbell and R.A. Anderson, "Effects of Aerobic Exercise and Training on the Trace

Minerals Chromium, Zinc, and Copper," <u>Sports Medicine</u> 4 (January-February 1987): 9-18.

5. "Fat-Burning Substances Can Assist Weight Loss," <u>Better Nutrition for Today's Living</u> 56 (June 1994), 13.

6. "Herbs, Like Drugs, Have a Dark Side," <u>Environmental Research</u> 16 (November 1993): 8.

7. "Nutrients Are Useful for Weight Reduction," <u>Better Nutrition for Today's Living</u> 54 (November 1992): 22.

## Chapter 5
## Calories—How High Can You Go?

1. Robyn Flipse, "The Dangers of Dieting Range from Dry Skin to Death: What to Do," <u>Environmental Nutrition</u> 14 (January 1991): 1-2.

2. "Fasting Isn't Faster," <u>Prevention</u> (September 1992): 29.

3. Janet Polivy, "Psychological Consequences of Food Restriction," <u>Journal of the American Dietetic Association</u> 96 (June 1996): 589-592.

4. Judith E. Brown, <u>The Science of Human Nutrition</u> (San Diego, California: Harcourt Brace Jovanovich, Publishers, 1990), 122 - 123.

5. Ibid.; Polivy, 589-592.

6. Polivy, 589-592.

7. L.A. Tucker and M. J. Kano, "Dietary Fat and Body Fat: A Multivariate Study of 205 Adult Females, <u>American Journal of Clinical Nutrition</u> 56 (October 1992): 616-622.

8. Wayne C. Miller, Michael G. Niederpruem, Janet P. Wallace, and Alice K. Lindeman, "Dietary Fat, Sugar, and Fiber Predict Body Fat Content," <u>Journal of the American Dietetic Association</u> 94 (June 1994): 612-615.

## Chapter 6
## Five Meals a Day

1. Maggie Spilner and Michele Stanten, "Automatic Weight Loss," <u>Prevention</u> (August 1996): 80-87.

## Chapter 7
## No More Hunger Pangs

1. N.A. King, V. J. Burley, and J. E. Blundell, "Exercise-induced Suppression of Appetite: Effects on Food Intake and Implications for Energy Balance," <u>European Journal of Clinical Nutrition</u> 48 (October 1994): 715-724; D. A. Thompson, L.

A. Wolfe, and R. Eikelboom, "Acute Effects of Exercise Intensity on Appetite in Young Men," <u>Medicine in Science and Sports Exercise</u> 20 (June 1988): 222-227.

## Chapter 8
## Fluids—What to Drink, What Not to Drink

1. Williams, 165.

2. Nancy Clark, "Fluid Facts: What, When, and How Much to Drink," <u>The Physician and Sportsmedicine</u> 20 (November 1992): 33-36.

3. Ibid.

4. Mark Tarnopolsky, "Protein, Caffeine, and Sports," <u>The Physician and Sportsmedicine 21</u> (March 1993): 137-146.

5. Michele Picozzi, "Drink Up," <u>Let's Live</u> (March 1996): 44-46.

6. Sue Browder, "Flatten Your Tummy Forever," <u>Reader's Digest</u> (June 1996), 80.

7. Eileen Mazer, "Natural Remedies for Fluid Retention," <u>Prevention</u> (December 1983): 106-112.

8. Ibid.

## Chapter 13
## Anti-Fat Exercise

1. R. Ross, H. Pedwell, and J. Rissanen, "Effects of Energy Restriction and Exercise on Skeletal Muscle and Adipose Tissue in Women as Measured by Magnetic Resonance Imaging," <u>American Journal of Clinical Nutrition</u> 61 (June 1995): 1179-1185.

2. University of Victoria, "Cycling Fat," <u>Canadian Journal of Sports Science</u>; 13: 204-207.

3. R. Bahr and O.M. Sejersted, "Effect of Intensity of Exercise on Excess Postexercise Oxygen Consumption," <u>Metabolism</u> 40 (August 1991): 836-841.

4. Candace Hogan, "Strength," <u>American Health</u> (November 1988): 55-59.

5. Judith E. Brown, <u>The Science of Human Nutrition</u> (San Diego, California: Harcourt Brace Jovanovich, Publishers, 1990), 78-82.

6. Judith Baker, "Resistance Training Basics: The What, Why and How of a Complete Fitness Program," <u>American Fitness</u> 12 (May-June 1994): 26-30.

## Chapter 14
## Choosing the Right Exercise

1. The Washington Post, "25 Percent of Americans Get No Daily Exercise," <u>Evansville Courier</u> (July 11, 1996): A-13.

**Chapter 15**
**Fat Loss Accelerators**
1. Chester J. Zelasko, "Exercise for Fat Loss: What Are the Facts?" <u>Journal of the American Dietetic Association</u> 95 (December 1995): 1414-1417.

**Chapter 18**
**Physique-Perfect Routines**
1. Thomas H. Maugh II, "A New Marker for Diabetes," <u>Science</u> 215 (February 1982): 651.
2. "Upper-Body Fat Distribution and Endometrial Cancer Risk," <u>Cancer Weekly</u> (October 14, 1991): 26-27; C.A. Swanson, N. Potischman, G. D. Wilbanks, L.B. Twiggs, et al, "Relation of Endometrial Cancer Risk to Past and Contemporary Body Size and Body Fat Distribution," <u>Cancer Epidemiology</u> 2 (July-August): 321-327.
3. "Upper-Body Fat Distribution and Endometrial Cancer Risk," 26-27.
4. "Adiposity, Fat Distribution and Cardiovascular Risk," <u>American Family Physician</u> 41 (March 1990): 962-963.
5. Bryant Stamford, "Apples and Pears," <u>The Physician and Sportsmedicine</u> 19 (January 1991): 123-124.
6. Ibid.
7. W. M. Kohrt, K. A. Obert, and J. O. Holloszy, "Exercise Training Improves Fat Distribution Patterns in 60 to 70-year-old Men and Women," <u>Journal of Gerontology</u> 47 (July 1992): M99-105.
8. M. S. Treuth, G. R. Hunter, T. Kekes-Szabo, R. L. Weinsier, et al, "Reduction in Intra-Abdominal Adipose Tissue after Strength Training in Older Women," <u>Journal of Applied Psychology</u> 78 (April 1995): 1425-1431.

**Chapter 19**
**The New You, Inside and Out**
1. Wire reports, "Umpire Granted Leave of Absence to Get in Shape," <u>Evansville Courier</u> (April 9, 1996): C2.
2. C. Everett Koop Foundation, "Shape Up America Report," 1995, 1.
3. Victoria, Moran, "Healthy, Wealthy, and Wise," <u>Ingram's</u> 20 (September 1994): 52-56.
4. Bonnie Liebman and David Schardt, "The Weighting Game," <u>Nutrition Action Healthletter</u> 22 (May 1995): 1-5.
5. William C. Rader, "Why Some Diets Don't Work," <u>Total Health</u> 16 (October 1994): 12-14.
6. Denise Foley, "Foods to Lower Your Blood Pressure," <u>Prevention</u> 36 (July 1984): 27-32.
7. Gail McBride, "Stroke: Our Hidden Health Risk," <u>Reader's Digest</u> (November 1996): 74-78.
8. M. W. Gillman, L. A. Cupples, D. Gagnon, B. M. Posner, R. C. Ellison, W. P. Castelli, and P. A. Wolf, "Protective Effect of Fruits and Vegetables on Development of Stroke in Men, " <u>JAMA</u> 273 (1995): 1113-1117.
9. C. Everett Koop Foundation, "Shape Up America Report," 1995, 12.
10. Ibid., 9-10.
11. Liebman and Schardt, 1-5.

**Chapter 20**
**Ever-After Lean**
1. Stephen Langer, "Nutritionally Coping with Stress," <u>Better Nutrition for Today's Living</u> 57 (July 1995): 42-44.

# Authors

**CLIFF SHEATS** is a clinical nutritionist and the creator and author of *Cliff Sheats' Lean Bodies* and *Cliff Sheats' Lean Bodies Total Fitness*, unique programs for losing body fat by following a nutritious, high-calorie eating program and an intense exercise program. Cliff is also the author of *The Lean Bodies Cookbook*.

He appears frequently as a guest expert on radio and television talk shows. In addition, he writes columns on nutrition for fitness publications, consults with amateur and professional athletes, and is involved in clinical research on nutrition.

Cliff is a certified clinical nutritionist. He has his bachelor of science degree in sports administration and nutrition, and his master of science degree in sports administration. He has worked in clinical practice with the medical profession (cardiology), specializing in nutrition. He is currently involved in a research Ph. D. program in London, England. Cliff is Fellow in Good Standing with the American Council of Applied Clinical Nutrition, a member of the International and American Associations of Clinical Nutritionists (IAACN), and member of the Royal Society of Health. Cliff is also a certified tennis professional with the United States Professional Tennis Registry USA.

**MAGGIE GREENWOOD-ROBINSON** is one of the country's best-known fitness authors. She is the co-author of seven other fitness books: *Cliff Sheats' Lean Bodies, Cliff Sheats' Lean Bodies Total Fitness, BUILT! The New Bodybuilding For Everyone, High-Performance Bodybuilding, John Parrillo's 50 Workout Secrets, High Performance Nutrition, and Shape Training: The 8-Week Total Body Makeover.*

Her articles have appeared in *Women's Sports and Fitness, Working Woman, Muscle and Fitness, Female Bodybuilding*, and many other publications. In addition, she has taught bodyshaping classes at the University of Southern Indiana. Maggie is currently working on a sports nutrition book for strength trainers.

**SWIMSUIT LEAN WORKOUT LOG**       Date:

**Resting Heart Rate:**              **Target Heart Rate:**

| EXERCISE | SETS/REPS | POUNDAGE |
|----------|-----------|----------|
|          |           |          |
|          |           |          |
|          |           |          |
|          |           |          |
|          |           |          |
|          |           |          |
|          |           |          |
|          |           |          |
|          |           |          |
|          |           |          |
|          |           |          |
|          |           |          |
|          |           |          |
|          |           |          |
|          |           |          |

| AEROBICS | TIME/DISTANCE | TIME OF DAY |
|----------|---------------|-------------|
|          |               |             |
|          |               |             |
|          |               |             |
|          |               |             |
|          |               |             |
|          |               |             |
|          |               |             |
|          |               |             |
|          |               |             |
|          |               |             |
|          |               |             |
|          |               |             |

## PERSONAL MENU PLANNER

**Date:**

| MEAL    FOODS | CALORIES |
|---|---|
| **Breakfast** | |
| | |
| | |
| | |
| | |
| | |
| | |
| | |
| **Mini/Mock Meal** | |
| | |
| | |
| **Lunch** | |
| | |
| | |
| | |
| | |
| | |
| | |
| | |
| **Mini/Mock Meal** | |
| | |
| | |
| **Dinner** | |
| | |
| | |
| | |
| | |
| | |
| | |
| | |
| | |
| | |

If you wish you may spread your calories over six meals a day instead of five. Just follow the aforementioned meal plans, but split up lunch or dinner to reach a total of six meals.

# Do you know about Lean Bodies classes?

## 1-800-697-LEAN

Eat more food...not less
and knock off body fat in the process!